Leadership in Nursing

Colleen Wedderburn Tate
President, CWT Enterprises;
Practising Midwife, career coach and mentor;
Associate, Centre for the Development of Nursing Practice and Policy, Leeds
University, UK

Foreword by

Beverly Alimo-Metcalfe PhD
Professor of Leadership Studies, University of Leeds,
Nuffield Institute for Health, Leeds, UK

Illustrations by Martin Davies

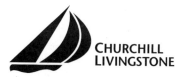

CHURCHILL
LIVINGSTONE

Edinburgh London New York Oxford Philadelphia St Louis Sydney Toronto 1999

CHURCHILL LIVINGSTONE
An imprint of Elsevier Limited

First published 1999
  Reprinted 2001, 2002, 2003, 2004

ISBN 0 443 06006 1

British Library Cataloguing in Publication Data
A catalogue record for this book is available from the British Library

Library of Congress Cataloging in Publication Data
A catalog record for this book is available from the Library of Congress

Note
Medical knowledge is constantly changing. As new information becomes
available, changes in treatment, procedures, equipment and the use of
drugs become necessary. The author and the publishers have, as far as it is
possible, taken care to ensure that the information given in this text is
accurate and up to date. However, readers are strongly advised to confirm
that the information, especially with regard to drug usage, complies with
the latest legislation and standards of practice.

The
publisher's
policy is to use
paper manufactured
from sustainable forests

Printed in China
B/05

Contents

Foreword

Never before has the need for leadership in organizations been so great – particularly in the National Health Service, which is so complex, so vast, so pressurized, and so important for the Nation's wellbeing.

Despite the plethora of literature that exists on leadership, or perhaps because of it, we need a book which provides a wealth of information on respected research in the topic, but which is also accessible, fun to read and highly practical. This is just such a book. For the reader who wishes to broaden or deepen their knowledge, this book also provides invaluable guidance.

If ever there was an individual who embodied the excitement, humanity and naturalness of transformational leadership, it would be for me Colleen Wedderburn Tate. Having experienced the fun of working with her, I have also learned much from her. Colleen 'tells it like it is', and in doing so she regularly 'shocks', but she does this with 'heart'.

She also affirms to those of us who passionately believe in its importance, that leadership is about being yourself and relishing the growth of others' leadership potential; accepting your and others' imperfections; celebrating your and others' differences but trying to do the best thing, which may often be somewhat challenging.

And this is the book's beauty. It is all about being and valuing 'you', and valuing and enabling others to be themselves, but always wanting to make things better.

I heartily recommend it to anyone who wants to change the world.

1999   Beverly Alimo-Metcalfe

Preface

This book was born out of a chance meeting at the Churchill Livingstone book stall at the 1996 RCN Congress. They were looking for a book on leadership, I was looking to write one. A marriage made in heaven.

This is a journey-man book (as in 'hard graft'). It is centred on the practice of leadership as experienced by me in a variety of settings, one of which is health care. I have written several articles on a variety of topics for healthcare, and other journals. Issues about leaders and leadership have been implicit in these articles, but not the central theme. But in preparing lectures for undergraduates and postgraduates, I was niggled by the emphasis on The Leader as almost a one-man (usually) band, single-handedly subduing nasty things called Bureaucracy, and Management, and The Way Things Are Done Around Here. I was niggled because the reality was so different from the books as to be almost extra-planetary.

The more I read, the more sceptical I became, and the more I recognized the same scepticism in colleagues. Not only were my nursing and midwifery colleagues unconvinced about the books, but nothing in their real experiences of their leaders led them to hope for better.

They saw unprincipled behaviour rewarded by promotion, saw expediency win out over principles, and were left to pick up the pieces. I dared to hope because if the NHS was really not capable of producing better leaders and better leadership, then we might as well all pack up and go home. What kept my scepticism under some control was the knowledge that I had known better in, and outside, the NHS.

And then there was *Star Trek*.

The more I watched the various *Star Trek* crews meet and greet more and more outlandish life forms, the more I was intrigued about the possibility that this series could be a template for a different kind of leader and leadership, one which explicitly depended on a group in order to succeed. What if the NHS in general, and nursing in particular, grew *Star Trek*-like captains, using situation analysis (see Chapter 3)? What if Lt Commander Data ran a hospital? What if the nurses fought for nursing the way the Bajorans fought the Cardassians – take no prisoners? What if all healthcare staff were shape-shifters, or coalescent beings (able to exactly reproduce any organic material they touched)? Would it change the price of eggs? Probably not, but at least it would get us talking in different ways about leaders and leadership.

As the 21st century comes tip-toeing into life, the debate about leaders and leadership becomes more intense. But with all this talk, who has time to lead? The trouble is, leaders make us feel uneasy. After all, they are lauded, rewarded, and accorded all kinds of powers. We 'ordinary people', who like nothing better than to see the powerful get their comeuppance, make suitably disgusted noises, while firmly denying that we have a hand in the events we so roundly criticize.

This book does not blame anyone for the failures of leadership that afflict health care. But I do insist that every healthcare worker has a responsibility to lead and exercise leadership. The fact that we may choose not to do so does not lessen our responsibility.

THE AUDIENCE

Although I focus on nurses and health care, this is not solely a book for nurse leaders. Anyone with an interest in talking and thinking about the topic is welcome to join in the conversation. No one is excluded, and no group should use any ideas in this book to bash others with.

HOW TO USE THIS BOOK

If you are one of those remarkable people who read a book, any book, systematically from Chapter 1 through to The End, fear not. You might find it difficult to find a logical story line, but you will get the gist nevertheless. For weirdos who start at the Index, then browse the first page of Chapter X, do a few of the exercises, then ignore the book for months, you will not be short changed either. Ideally, this is a book to reflect on. It is also one you can leave open at 'certain pages' to make a point to someone.

I make no apology for limiting pure theory to one chapter. Again, we theorize so much about leadership that we have no puff left to actually do it. You will find many theories winding their way through this book. None of them is infallible. I have put my own interpretation on these theories to make sense of my experience of being led, and of being a leader. Feel free to do the same.

Write your own stories about leaders and leadership. We need to hear different voices on this topic, not just the 'acknowledged authorities'. Also at issue is the fact that the voice of leadership, at least in the text books, is still dominantly male. Women talk about leadership, and do it, in different ways to men, and I speak about this a lot in the book. Neither is right nor wrong, just different.

CONTENT AND STYLE

The book is written as if you and I are having a conversation about leadership. I am not keen on one-sided conversations, but in this case an exception can be made. I chose the conversational style because I feel that it is less stilted, and is perfect for story-telling, a form of research which I value, and which is much under-rated in health care. Our conversation takes place over 12 chapters, book-ended by this preamble and a 'So What?' end-piece, a *mea culpa*.

In Chapter 1, our conversation starts with a look at this thing called leadership, concentrating on why people choose to lead, what happens when we make these choices inappropriately, and the fall-out from forgetting about ethics and emotions. Chapter 2 relates six stories of leaders who have had an impact on my life.

In Chapters 3 and 4 we talk about the theory and practice of leadership, teasing out how nurses can become more proactive leaders. Chapter 5 is very personal to you, and uses quizzes based on what we talk about in Chapters 2 and 4. In Chapters 4 and 5 we play 'spot the leader', what these people do and do not know about themselves.

For the next four chapters, our conversation is partly philosophical, and mainly nitty-gritty. How do we create better leaders? How will we know when we are better leaders? Why do leaders fail? Chapter 10 reveals the Cardinal Sins of leadership, while in Chapter 11, we speculate about nurses and leadership in the 21st century. What will nurses need to do, and know, to successfully lead health care? Who will be the main supporters of what nurses want to achieve as leaders?

Leaders who exist outside the corporate model of leadership, which is the standard against which leaders are judged, are the focus of Chapter 12. For several years I have been examining and observing non-corporate models of leadership. Max de Pree calls it 'leadership without power'. This concept will be familiar to people who are involved in community participation projects. For nurses, non-corporate types of leadership need to be understood because that's how the communities we work with operate.

This is just the beginning of our conversation. I would like to know what you think about what we talk about in this book. Meanwhile, I will continue to read and write about leaders and leadership, ponder wacky ideas from *Star Trek*, and always aim to follow the maxim: If not now, when? If not me, who?

If you have been, thanks for listening.

1999   C.W.T.

Acknowledgements

Thanks to Alex Mathieson, who planted the idea and fixed my attention on it; to the leaders who have taught me how to and how not to; to my partner, Clive, who is the most picky editor I have ever met and who did not badger to read every chapter.

Thanks also to Martin Davies, the people who write about leadership and those who talk with me about it, and who do it with such panache and grace.

I would also like to thank Beverly Alimo-Metcalfe for being an inspiration in how she speaks, acts and writes leadership.

Leaders R us

Key words:

choices; dilemmas; Reality Checklist; transformational leadership;
success; failure

Leadership is not about promotion to a senior job, or preparing for one. If that's your view, this book will disappoint you.

Remember the days in the playground, when Miss Bossy Boots, or her alter ego, Mr Take Charge, made life hell? This book is about what happens when those first experiences of leadership get mixed with theories about leadership, causing distorted ideas about who leaders are, and what they do.

Take a long look around the organization for which you work. It may be painfully clear that the adult world is not a playground. As children, most of us were very good at playing, having fun, dreaming, being optimistic, and generally feeling hopeful about the future. Before we became employees, we were relatively free spirits. In becoming employees, some of us have lost that part of ourselves which knew how to have fun.

So here you and I sit, tentatively beginning a dialogue about leadership and leading. Whatever your reason for being here, mine is simple: to help you to recognize that leadership and leading are accessible to everyone – at a price. At the end of our dialogue, you may decide that leadership is too hard, too demanding, too exhausting, and you might feel it is not for you. Alternatively, you may decide that it is the most fun you can have while sober. Whatever you choose, we will at least have had the opportunity to think about, and discuss in depth, a subject that is too often treated superficially, drowned in jargon, and made irrelevant to everyday nursing practice.

DO YOU KNOW THE WAY TO SAN JOSÉ?

Let me give you an example. At a meeting of clinical nurse specialists I attended, the results from a survey on patients' opinions about the pain relief they received after surgery were presented. Half-way through the meeting, it became clear that a nurse-led pain management unit was likely to provide the most effective solution to meeting the patients' expressed needs. There was certainly no money within the hospital to fund such a unit, and little enthusiasm from some medical staff to support a nurse-led project.

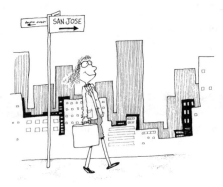

Do you know the way?

By the end of the meeting, the nurse specialists decided to seek funding for a pain management unit from a drug company, or other source. This might seem a perfectly logical, if not startlingly obvious, conclusion. But it was the ease with which everyone at the meeting was reconciled to *not* finding the money for a new unit *internally* which startled me so much. Some people expressed discomfort with the notion of a drug company funding the set-up of a pain management unit (again, no surprises there), but the lack of support from medical and management colleagues for an *internal* solution to the problem was never discussed – it was simply assumed, and accepted.

There were several consequences of this outcome:

- The clinical nurse specialists continue to have little influence over resource decisions.
- Doctors and managers in the hospital believe that nurses have interest in, but little power to challenge, spending decisions.
- Junior nursing staff continue to be frustrated at the lack of nursing leadership in pushing for improvements in patient care and in the promotion of nursing.
- Nurse-led projects are not a priority at the hospital.

It is easy to point the finger at senior nurse colleagues who, we may feel, have not done as much as they could to keep patients at the centre of health service priorities. We know the stark choices we face as buyers, providers and users of health care. We also know the price of having to make those choices. It's important, therefore, to take a critical look at how we use leadership to advance patient care, to develop nursing practice, and to transform our health service organizations. This is more difficult than the easy task of finding scapegoats.

CHOICES AND DILEMMAS

Over the past decade or so, the shelf life of a leader in the health service has probably halved. Instead of working in an environment that encourages creative thinking about the future of health care, we have one which consists of vast paper trails, characterized by random motion masquerading as activity. Stand-up comics lampoon us for being in endless meetings about meetings. The 'luxury' of a personal life for senior staff is frowned upon in some healthcare organizations, and 60-hour working weeks are quite normal.

Some healthcare staff are no longer working for patients, but are more motivated by pronouncements from government ministers, exposés in the media, and the latest scandal about misuse of public money. Different parts of healthcare organizations seem to focus on different things, with poor coordination across departments. There seems, for example, little dove-tailing between drives to keep costs down, and efforts to increase patient services. Even the much-maligned hospital administrators feel the cutting edge of this incoordination; at a time when demands for administrative services are increasing, administrative jobs are being cut.

Making choices requires a certain amount of freedom of thought and action, some time to weigh the options, and time to review the decision made. In health care, leaders have few of these luxuries. The reliable, relevant and easily accessible information they need to make decisions is frequently not available; even if it was, the resources and time to make use of it are missing. Much of what healthcare leaders do is driven by gut feeling, linked to a strong sense of personal values about what is right, reasonable, and just. That may be the only focal point that a leader, intent on making a success of the job, has in an uncertain environment.

Irrespective of what country they operate in, healthcare leaders fulfil several roles – diplomat, visionary, conflict resolver, politician, figurehead, coach, and human being. If you believe the books, no leader today can lay claim to the title unless she or he does all of the above, and becomes a motivational speaker to boot. Where is the time to think about the future, and not just pontificate about it? Where is the support system they need to do all this heroic stuff? What about the little, quiet things, like remembering a colleague's birthday, gossiping, talking with patients and relatives, going to lunch before it is time to go home?

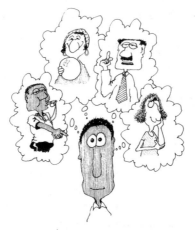

Multiple personality

Undeniably, some of the pressures leaders face concern sharing a little piece of themselves with anyone that asks. But healthcare leaders, like others, face real dilemmas.

How can they:

- radically change their organization, without any guarantee of success, no matter how well the change is planned, and accept the consequences?
- work with political agendas or legislation they disagree with, and accept the consequences?
- apportion scarce resources as fairly as possible, and accept the consequences?
- say 'no' when they want to say 'yes', and accept the consequences?
- always try to act ethically, and sometimes fail?
- know that, no matter what they do, someone, somewhere will cry 'foul'?

They also have to make choices. For example, they have to decide whether to:

- always act on absolute principles, or create several flexible responses
- keep particular services, or discard them
- have an open organization – always, sometimes, or never
- develop closer ties with services users, but have little control over the eventual outcome
- continue to lead, or not.

This book attempts to help you face such dilemmas and make choices, even in the face of seemingly overwhelming odds. *Not* choosing is also a choice, and can be a positive response in the short term. It buys thinking time. But in the long term, doing nothing turns choices into dilemmas, and ultimately the leader who delays making a choice might have to opt for the better of two bad alternatives.

FOCUSED ACTION

The essence of leadership is focused action. Acting on the evidence before you is all you need to do, but action can be paralyzed by any number of considerations, including concern for one's own reputation and status (see Box 1.1 for an example of this).

Box 1.1   Case

A young woman was admitted to a hospital ward with a suspected deep vein thrombosis (DVT). An infusion, by pump, of heparin was started, and an X-ray ordered. The standing guidelines for the treatment of suspected DVT were:

- heparin 45,000 IU, by pump, 12 hourly, for a maximum of 48 hours
- X-ray within 24 hours to confirm diagnosis
- prothrombin times to be done daily while heparin infusion continues
- bed rest, except for toileting purposes
- review patient daily, or at any time if condition changes.

On several occasions, the woman asked how long the infusion would last, and when she would be going home. She was told that the infusion would come down 'soon'.

Five days after her admission, an agency nurse read in the woman's notes that an X-ray had been requested to be done on the day after admission. This had not happened. Prothrombin times had not been done for 3 days, the last sample having clotted. The heparin infusion continued.

The ward manager to whom this was reported explained that she had called the X-ray department about an appointment for the woman on numerous occasions, with no success.

At the end of 6 days, the woman's consultant became aware of these circumstances when he requested, and did not get, the X-rays. When asked about the X-rays, the ward-based staff argued that 'X-ray said they were busy'.

The agency nurse, who had been a senior clinical nurse before taking early retirement, had suggested calling the consultant radiologist directly, and also informing the nurse manager in charge of the unit. The ward manager had responded: 'If I did that, they would say I can't cope'.

The woman in the case in Box 1.1 suffered no lasting harm from her admission. But the ward manager's fear of being labelled 'unable to cope' prevented her from acting in this patient's best interests. You may ask: 'is a patient's best interest worth my reputation, or even my job?' For some, the answer has been (and may continue to be) 'yes'. In this case, the ward manager and her staff had clear guidelines to use as a lever for action, but even if there had been no guidelines, there would still have been scope for action. The commonsense recognition that patients with unconfirmed diagnoses merit regular review would have been a starter. As a minimum, the woman's questions about her condition demanded the action of giving accurate information.

Failure to act in part of a decision may lead to general inaction. In the example in Box 1.1, the lack of nursing and medical action on reviewing the treatment requested on admission, led to inaction on delivering treatment. The ward manager's pivotal leadership role was overshadowed by fear of unjust criticism. If you find yourself delaying decisions, despite evidence that you have to act quickly, the ultimate consequences for you are guilt, and a sense of failure.

NOTHING SUCCEEDS LIKE FAILURE

Leaders fail when they do not consider the consequences of choosing. The greater the impact of the action, the more careful the leader must be in the choices she or he makes. For example, it is flattering to be invited to take charge of a prestigious project. But it is unwise not to have an internal conversation with yourself, when you can be free to admit that you have no idea how to deliver the desired outcome. This internal conversation serves as a check against overindulgence in hubris. It may also prevent harm befalling others, and yourself.

We presume that, as leaders, others will willingly follow us. But to have any chance of earning such a privilege, we need to stand back, sit still, and reflect on the kind of person we are. Only then can we begin to make sense of what leadership is, and can be.

The ward manager in the example in Box 1.1 may want to take issue with this. In the over-tasked world that is nursing care, there is little enough time to care for patients, much less for the luxury of taking time out to think and reflect. But time for reflection is a necessity, not a luxury. When we are not clear about why we do things, we create the conditions for needless failure. It is difficult enough to succeed when we have goals. It is twice as tough when we have little direction, and do not take the time to think about how we do our work.

The most effective people and leaders I have worked with have spent several years in a personal inquiry, clarifying their core values to themselves. This is often an uncomfortable process, but a necessary one. Such people accept the risks involved in leading because they have made a free choice to be a leader. They have not viewed leadership as a way to get promotion, or gain exaggerated (or unjustified) praise. Getting to know yourself inside out is not 'touchy feely'. It is just about the only way to stay sane and productive. As Helen Keller said: 'I do not want the peace that passeth understanding. I want the understanding that bringeth peace' (Warner 1992).

Failure is one consequence of inattention to what makes us tick, and it can be fatal – to our self-esteem, self-confidence, sense of worth, and sense of self. As nurses, we often fail to forgive failure in ourselves and others. If we can picture failure as a step on the continuum to success, however, we can learn not to repeat the same mistake. Admittedly, in health care, failure can have serious consequences, but even these failures are occasions for learning, as I know from personal experience. Prevention most certainly *is* better than cure.

So, how do you handle failure? If you have chosen to be a leader, then you will already know that not succeeding 100% every time is part of the job description. If you have stumbled into leadership, and have not talked through, with yourself, your fears and uncertainties, failure will always be an unwelcome surprise.

WHAT'S IN IT FOR ME? – OR THE *WIIFM* FACTOR IN LEADERSHIP

If leadership is not about job promotion, why do it? Frankly, I like leading things because people get to see how good I can be, and so do I. On the other hand, there are some occasions when I like to keep my light under the most dense bush – the occasions when I have no idea what is going on, do not really care, and would rather read a good book.

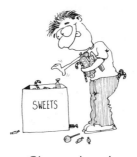

Gimme, gimme!

I freely confess that my pragmatic attitude to leadership has not brought universal acclaim. At least one person has labelled it the 'only-when-I-want-to' syndrome. But that is exactly my point. We need to be sure of the right time to stick our necks out, take a stand on some principle, drive some idea or change, or just go a different road to everyone else. And we need to be sure *why* we are prepared to do it. If we are not clear and honest with ourselves and others about why we want to become a leader, we will simply store up problems for everyone – ourselves most definitely included.

Over time, I have developed a Reality Checklist of questions I use in times of great self-confidence – when I am feeling particularly sure that I know exactly what I am doing, and where I am going. I use the Reality Checklist in several ways:

- as a means of taking time-out to think
- as an aid to making decisions I would rather avoid, but can't
- for self-development, in association with self-assessment inventories (more on these later)
- to assist in coaching sessions
- to confirm decisions.

I find that using the Reality Checklist guards against hubris and general self-delusion, helps me keep a sense of proportion, and enables me to focus on what is important. The Reality Checklist follows.

Reality Checklist

1. If I were guaranteed success in anything I chose to do, what one thing would I spend the rest of my life doing?

2. Which person has been most influential in my life? (parents/family members are included).

3. What is my most precious possession?

4. If I won the lottery or the pools, what are the first three things I would do?

5. What is the most memorable thing that has ever happened to me?

6. What makes me angry?

7. What makes me sad?

8. What makes me cry?

9. What gives me the most enjoyment?

10. What is my worst fault?

11. What is my best trait?

12. What is my greatest fear?

13. Who am I, really?

If you would like to, try the Reality Checklist now, taking note of the comments above. It is not something to be done in a hurry – you will need about 2 hours. If you are not used to spending time on your own, talking with yourself, you may still be on the first question at the end of the time. Don't worry. Take it step by step, asking the questions in no particular order. The only stipulation is that you be honest with your answers, because no one is checking up on you. Remember that the purpose of the exercise is to help to keep you focused in times of stress or confusion. Make a note of your answers if you prefer, but don't beat yourself up if you don't give yourself the answer you think you should. Being honest is more important than getting perfect scores.

I used to make a note of all the answers I made, and would get very anxious if I found I had different answers to the same questions over time. Now that I take myself much less seriously, the answers matter less. More important is the process of reflection, and dreaming, that the Reality Checklist facilitates. The sense of having some control over what you do, and how you act, is a powerful source of a leader's ability to be effective, and enables her or him to function under stress. There will be more time to study and use the checklist when we look at the characteristics of effective leaders later in the book.

So, 'what's in it for me?' Some leaders crave public recognition. Some crave love, some respect. Others crave glory. Fine. As long as we admit to ourselves that this is what we are about.

You and I can sit here and count the number of our colleagues we consider to be leaders – the people who can help us do better than we ever dreamed. We also know others who have the title of leader. Committed and highly qualified people as they are, they are not attached to what they do. They lead because it is in the job description. We are not interested in such leaders-because-of-title. Our business is with the other kind: leader-because-I-choose-to-be.

In so many organizations, leadership is assumed to be the role of those at the top. What we forget is that when we are at the top, we cannot lead anything without first finding ways to connect to the rest of the organization. The effects of not doing so can be devastating for everyone in the organization.

Take, as an example, the board of a manufacturing company who called in an experienced management consultant to help them find out why their staff were disaffected, unhappy, and increasingly belligerent. After hearing from board members how apathetic the staff were, how uncooperative, how lacking in motivation, and how they did not have the interest of the company at heart, the consultant asked if the board had shared the company's vision statement with the staff. The chief executive explained that the vision statement was for the board, and not for the workers. All that was required of them was to trust the judgment of the company's leaders, and get on with it.

Of course, such styles of leadership are not exclusive to the world of big business. They are not difficult to find in the health services. Consider, for example, the story of the senior managers in an acute hospital who decided to close some wards over the Christmas period. This seemed perfectly sensible, because hospital policy was to try to discharge as many patients as possible during this period. In this case, though, the wards chosen for temporary closure were care of the elderly wards.

As chance would have it, it turned out to be a particularly severe winter. Ambulances began bringing injured and ill elderly people in to casualty, with nowhere to admit them. As it was Christmas, social services' cover was minimal. Accident and emergency, medical staff, the nursing director, general practitioners, ward staff, the ambulance centre, catering staff – none had been consulted before the decision on closure was made. It is pretty safe to assume that if they had, a different decision would have been reached.

Admittedly, this is an extreme example. But I wonder how many times decisions have been taken in your hospital 'at the top' with little discussion with the people who have to implement the decision? And how many times have we, as nurses, taken decisions which affect the care of a patient, without involving her or him in the process?

There are probably many organizations where some staff are uninterested in the longterm future of the business, do their required hours each day, and go home. But lack of interest in the future of an organization is not the same as not caring about it, if only because money from the job pays the bills. Effective leaders do not always have the perfect staff, the perfect job, the perfect life, nor are they necessarily perfect people. But they know that sloppy leadership equals sloppy followership.

Most of us want to do it right. We know it is right to talk to our colleagues honestly, openly, and not treat them as if they are stupid. After all, we all want to be treated like intelligent beings. So how come, when we are in the driving seat, it can turn out so differently? It is not that we are bad, or evil (although there has been the odd case of leaders victimizing the led). No, we are sincere in what we do. And we mean to do it right. It is just that some days, we can get distracted from doing what is right.

TAKE ME AWAY FROM IT ALL

Sometimes we forget that we are human first, and everything else after that. Just think of the many times when you just wanted to give it all up, and let someone else make all the decisions for you. The times when you felt it was easier to stifle your objections than take a stand. When you did not act in the right way, and bit off the head of the person who told you so.

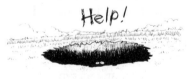

Rescue me

And it is OK to feel all those things. Go back to the Reality Checklist. Nothing on that list presumes that we are superhuman. On the contrary, leadership is to be fully human, with all our frailties and ... derstandable that some of us expect our leaders to be better ... why should we?

... mes you have faced almost crippling uncertainty within ... ll found some source of strength, something which pushed ... of your fears. It can be very comforting to read about peo- ... overcome terrible odds. But the biggest odds you can ever overcome is the fear of not being able to cope. The penultimate question on the Reality Checklist is: What is my greatest fear? I don't know about you, but one of mine (only one!) is not being able to even ask that question. Attachment to her or his humanity is what marks out a great leader.

ETHICS AND EMOTION IN LEADERSHIP – TRANSFORMATIONAL LEADERSHIP OR 'EATING ELEPHANTS'

Writers on transformational leadership, which we will discuss in more detail later, tell us that it is transformational leaders' emotional attachment to the people and issues they lead which makes them stand out.

Transformational leaders want to know what makes people tick. They are interested in what people do, what they want to achieve from the work they do, how they want to contribute to the organization, and how they can help others. They still do the business of setting and meeting targets, managing the money, assigning responsibility, and being accountable. But they get the job done by getting others to 'eat elephants'. Let me explain.

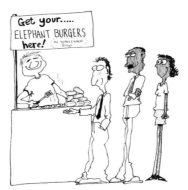

Elephant burgers

'Elephant' is an analogy for those tasks that leaders have to do (as in 'elephantine task'). The term can also be used to describe large organizations whose traditional 'elephantine' structures make it difficult for them to respond to change. It is difficult to eat an 'elephant' in one, or even several, sittings. What we have to do is cut it into manageable, digestible, 'elephant burgers'.

When you think about it, this makes sense. Work is hard enough without indigestion as a regular part of the day. Transformational leaders know how many elephants there are to be eaten. They also know that there may be many others just over the horizon. They take advice from people who are expert elephant spotters (that is, anyone). The leader works through them to decide the best way to cut the elephant into burgers. This doesn't mean that the leader abandons accountability for tracking where the elephants are, or are likely to come from. But sharing the decisions gives more options, with a greater possibility that, should elephants arise from an unexpected quarter, there is scope to deal with them.

While doing all this, transformational leaders must always act ethically. Manipulating and undermining others, being deliberately misleading, believing 'the ends justifies the means', and not recognizing right from wrong, are not part of the process of accomplishing objectives. Because a leader's role is to achieve the task, maintain relationships, and treat individuals with respect, transformational leaders work within a strong ethical framework.

My first experience of a transformational leader was unsettling. This man wanted me to tell him what he could do to make my job easier. This completely threw me. He was the BOSS, for heaven's sake. But I am an opportunist and I took the bait. We had a detailed and honest discussion about my future, the possible direction of the organization, and how I had contributed to helping him do his job.

I shall never forget that afternoon. He listened, actively, while I talked (I still speak to him occasionally, and that quality of listening is always present), and I found I was attending to how he responded, verbally and nonverbally, to what I said. This meant that I became focused on thinking before I spoke. Instead of my usual stream-of-consciousness outflow, I had to think clearly about the work I was doing and wanted to do, how I wanted to structure my work-time to allow me some life-time, and how I should articulate my views. At no time during our 2-hour meeting did I feel that he was in a hurry to be somewhere else.

All of our one-to-one meetings had this clarity, and staff meetings were similarly transformed. He always took the Any Other Business (AOB) item first. He believed this helped people concentrate on the business of the meeting, rather than worrying that there would not be enough time at the end to speak about something important to them. Interesting that after the change was implemented, few AOB items involved anything more than information sharing; the days of tabling a 20-page document in the last 5 minutes of the staff meeting were history.

Since then, I have been privileged to work with more transformational leaders. Like love, once you have experienced the real thing, nothing less will do. But what if you do not have a boss like that? Health care is full of less-than transforming managers-with-leader-in-their-title. But maybe you have a friend or colleague who has the rare ability to focus on what you are saying (and not saying) and can help you to think (and listen) more clearly. Maybe you have that ability, and can enable others to learn from you.

Leaders in the making (not those on the make) view every experience as an opportunity for learning, about themselves, other people, or things. Leadership is not about promotion to a senior job, or preparing for one. Leaders cannot get the best from the people who choose to follow them unless there is some attachment between them, an attachment not specified in the contract of employment.

You may worry that taking a transformational approach to leadership may lead to other people taking advantage of you. And that may happen. That is why leadership is a choice. Shutting down the capacity to be hurt hinders our ability to recognize hurt in others. It also hinders our capacity to heal, and move on.

To lead effectively is to be fully human, and that will probably involve pain of some kind. But after the pain, comes the joy. Just like plants, we need winters to harden us, and prepare us for the fun of spring and summer. If you want to be an effective leader, there is a lot of rough with the smooth. But the smooth is worth the wait.

Transformational leadership is becoming the model of leadership in many organizations, especially those in competition for more market-share for their products. Healthcare and social care organizations are also beginning to take notice. We have an increasingly demanding clientele, and not just for services. Healthcare users expect to be treated with dignity, courtesy, and respect. They may not say this in so many words, but the yearly reports from the Health Service Ombudsman show that the single biggest category of patient complaints about the NHS is poor communication, between staff, and from staff to patients. This is odd, given that providing health care is an intensely interactive process. But it is also emotionally taxing, and can lead to a willingness to limit communication with each other, with patients, and with relatives.

Transformational leaders should, by definition, be numerous in health care. Apparently, they are not. Hypnotized by heroic tales from the commercial sector, aggressive management, as opposed to effective leadership, remains the norm. 'Action Manager' is seemingly preferable to 'Thoughtful Leader', who puts brain into gear before speaking. The current environment of our healthcare system – finance-driven, short-term initiatives, territorial battles, intolerance of differing opinions – is not conducive to producing transformational leaders. Yet they are beginning to reveal themselves at ward level, where the ethos remains focused on patient care. These emergent leaders know their limitations, and their possibilities. They may work in hostile environments, but ultimately they make a success of what they do by supporting each other.

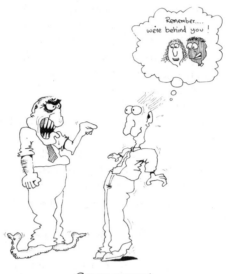

Group support

Picture this. You spend a day revamping a job description and place an advertisement for a 'person with excellent interpersonal skills', among other attributes. You talk to several interested applicants. You arrange a day or two of interviews and meetings. You organize a 3-week induction programme and fix up the new appointee with all the trappings that go with the job. This person really believes in the organization's aims and objectives, and is clear that working for you will be in harmony with her own values. Less than 6 months later, she resigns.

Why? It is tempting to say 'she didn't fit in'. Maybe so, but if she fitted 6 months ago, why not now? What caused such a dramatic change? Could the fault lie with the organization?

In a 1997 report, the Audit Commission stated that 'good or bad managers are a bigger cause of the variation in staff turnover [in the NHS] … than all other factors put together' (Audit Commission 1997). Put another way, a student nurse once remarked to me: 'I came into nursing as a person. I am now a thing, and am treated as such.' Almost every week, the health-care press carries stories about instances of poor management – lack of consultation on changes, bullying, discrimination, and lack of common courtesy. Many organizations treat their employees less than perfectly. In health care, the least we should expect is that we treat each other with a minimum of regard. It is very hard to plan a fight against a herd of elephants when some of the defendants are in their own private war.

Leadership can be emotionally exhausting, and creates ethical conflicts concerning how and when to act. This is part of learning to be an effective leader, and there are few short cuts. But leadership carries fringe benefits.

ADVANTAGES OF LEADERSHIP

Imagine being able to do anything you want – as long as other people believed in you enough to help you. Imagine being able to help others to realize their goals, and they have no idea that you have helped them. Imagine the pain of spectacular failure, and the joy of knowing you need never make the same mistake again – at least not in the same way.

Then there are the tangible rewards – recognition by peers, fame, money, awards. The most extreme tangible rewards appear to accrue to those leaders who are viewed as heroes, such as bosses of large commercial companies or political leaders. But nurses are also given recognition for being leaders – The RCN/*Nursing Standard* Nurse of the Year, the *Nursing Times*/3M Awards, sponsored scholarships, fellowships, access to professional development opportunities.

Ultimately, however, leadership is its own reward. There is personal pride in enabling others to reach their optimum potential. Satisfaction in effecting change. The elation that you did what you may have thought was beyond your capability. For me, the main advantage of being a leader is the

Key learning points

- Leadership is not about promotion.

- Leaders choose to lead.

- If leaders do not know why they want to lead, they may make unnecessary mistakes, sometimes with harmful consequences.

- Leaders need to make regular reality checks to prevent arrogance and complacency getting in the way of their effectiveness.

- The most effective leaders adopt a transformational style which emphasizes emotional connection to the goal, and ethical behaviour.

- It is helpful for leaders to find out the different methods of 'eating elephants'.

- Leadership has advantages, the least of which is the ability to be optimally effective and productive.

- Leaders are *us*.

sense of having created something against the odds. That kind of high is the impetus for further achievement, always with the caveat that next time, it may not happen that way.

REFERENCE

Warner C 1992 The last word: a treasury of womens' quotes. Prentice Hall, Hemel Hempstead, p 224

Born to lead?

Key words:

stories; commitment; effective leadership

Some writers on leadership say that leaders are ordinary people who do extraordinary things (Kouzes & Posner 1995, Peters & Waterman 1995). Others argue that leadership is an art learned over time (De Pree 1989), and that leaders are effective users of power (Moss Kanter 1977). People who write about and study leaders can help us understand more clearly the characteristics that define effective leaders.

In Chapter 3, we will look at various theories of leadership and how they have changed over time. In Chapter 5, we will discuss in detail the characteristics of effective leaders, using Kouzes and Posner's work. For now, let's focus on six people who, while not all famous, are leaders. Their stories show leadership in action, and bring dry theory to life.

No doubt you have your own stories to tell about people who have made leadership alive for you. I have chosen these six people because they represent for me the essence of leadership – seeing something that has to be fixed, and fixing it.

They range from a nurse to a factory owner. They are also from different centuries. The issues they faced are recognizable, and are still around today – changing unfair systems, tackling ill-health in a vulnerable community, changing clinical practice, dealing with catastrophic emergencies.

Two of the stories are well known – those of Mary Seacole and Aaron Feuerstein (their real names). One, Lynda Randolph, is a national figure in her own country. The others are known only to their local community. But they have lots in common:

- courage
- determination
- commitment to what they set out to do
- patience in the face of obstacles
- a desire to make things better.

As you read their stories, think about the things you may want to change at work, or elsewhere. How determined are you? Are you committed to doing whatever it takes to make the change? Are you willing to accept the consequences of fighting for that change? How you answer those questions is probably less important than having the courage to ask them in the first place.

Remember that leaders often emerge because of prevailing circumstances. The six people are, or were, of their time, but how they approached their work is still relevant today. Now, the stories.

WILLING TO SERVE – MARY JANE SEACOLE

Among the many stories of leaders and leadership, Mary Seacole's stands out for several reasons. She was, among other things:

- a black woman making her own living and her own way in the 19th century
- an acute observer of the influence of the USA in Latin America
- a doctress (female healer with medical knowledge) who used her skills to treat infectious diseases
- a gold prospector
- a woman who viewed life as an adventure.

Mary Seacole tells her story better than anyone, and you can read her autobiography, first published in 1857 and re-issued in 1984 (Alexander & Dewjee 1984). My aim is to show how, when you are determined to do something, not much can stand in your way.

Mary Seacole was born in Jamaica in 1805, the daughter of a black mother and white Scottish army officer father; she was therefore a mulatto (person of mixed race). Her mother ran a boarding house which was frequented by naval and army officers and their families.

Her early years were influenced by the military attitudes of the people who boarded with her mother, and were overshadowed by slavery. She was free-born and, by the standards of the day, well-off. Mulattos tended to be well-educated, as many Jamaican planters sent their black children to be schooled in Europe. But in common with all free black people, mulattos had few civil rights: no vote, barred from entering the professions and from holding public office, and limited in the amount of money they could inherit.

From an early age, Mary loved to travel. Before her marriage to Edward Horatio Seacole (Horatio Nelson's godson), she had twice travelled to England and had visited Cuba, the Bahamas, and Haiti. In those days, travel was long and tedious, but Mary was adventurous, a spirit which led her to live in Panama and to work on the battlefield in the Crimean War. It is for this work that Mary Seacole is best known.

She was a contemporary of Florence Nightingale who, by some accounts, thought highly of her, although the two women never met. Mary travelled to England to volunteer to go to the Crimea with Nightingale's group of nurses. She felt that her experience of treating soldiers with cholera in Panama would be very useful in the Crimea, where similar conditions prevailed.

Turned down for service because of her age (she was in late middle-age) and colour ('I read in [one of Miss Nightingale's companion's] face, that had there been a vacancy, I should not have been chosen to fill it', she wrote), Mary bought her own supplies and travelled to the Crimea as a sutler (someone who sells goods to soldiers). She printed a set of cards and sent them to her friends in Sebastopol, announcing her arrival at Balaclava 'to establish a mess-table and comfortable quarters for sick and convalescent soliders'. She set up her *British Hotel* on the battlefield, and nursed, fed, bandaged, and generally cared for thousands of soldiers.

The Crimean War ended abruptly in 1856, leaving Mary with expensive (and redundant) stock. By November that year she was in the bankruptcy court, but with the help of her many friends in England, all her debts were discharged by February 1857. Her friends also raised funds to 'place her beyond the reach of want'. For the remainder of her life, she lived between Jamaica and England. She died a relatively wealthy woman in May 1881.

What drew this small, middle-aged 'yellow' woman (as she called herself) to the horrors of the Crimea? In her autobiography, Mary describes her longing to go to Russia, partly to witness the war, and partly because many of the regiments she had know in Jamaica were there. She also vividly relates her struggle to obtain official permission to travel to the Crimea. What would have been the final straw in terms of rejection for most people simply made Mary more determined.

Mary Seacole's life was lived at a pace that many of us would find exhausting. She relished challenges, more so if they involved serving others. She was determined in whatever she did, even if she had to make all the running. I doubt if she ever fully appreciated her leadership qualities. Few leaders do, being so busy making things better.

Mary comes to mind every time I face what looks like an insurmountable obstacle, an equivalent Crimea. She lived her life up to and beyond the edge. We do not have to be exactly like her to have the same impact, but her story shows that effective leaders, from whatever century and whatever country, are fundamentally alike in their willingness to take risks to achieve their goals.

A ROOM IS NOT A HOME – ANNE SMITH

Meet Anne Smith (not her real name). At the time her story begins, she is a 19-year-old student nurse in the 1970s. She lives in the nurses' home attached to the hospital where she is taking her 3-year training.

Anne's parental home was not in the UK. For the first year of her training, she had no family in the UK. She made several strong friendships among the other resident nurse students, and they formed her family group. Anne had not planned on being a nurse. Family tragedy had changed her intention of becoming a doctor. But she was always able to turn any situation into an opportunity, and settled into the UK (and the nursing school) without too many problems. Except for one thing.

In those days, nurses' homes were run and managed by a home warden. Usually retired nurses, the wardens were like surrogate mothers. A nurses' home full of high energy young women, who were dealing with life and death issues every day, produced, naturally, a boisterous atmosphere. Many wardens saw it as their duty to keep this energy under control.

There was no harsh discipline in Anne's nurses' home, but there were rules, one of which was that nurses were not allowed to have male friends visit them in the home. This rule was established primarily to prevent nurses taking male friends up to their rooms. Breaking the rule meant a visit to the matron's office, a conversation between the matron and your parents, and possible expulsion from the home.

Anne had thought this rule unfair. It was sometimes used to break up what the warden saw as 'unsuitable relationships'. She also used the rule as justification to carry out searches of students' rooms in their absence, and 'check up' on them. On one such occasion, Anne was in her room when the warden entered, unannounced. Angry and embarrassed, Anne challenged the warden to justify her actions.

After she left, Anne decided that she could not live under such conditions. Her own home was a warm, forgiving place. For the first time since she arrived, she wanted to give up and leave nursing and the UK. A short telephone call to her mother put things into perspective.

Her sister and brother-in-law had recently arrived in the UK and were living in London. One weekend in early winter, they visited Anne. After taking them to lunch in a local restaurant, she brought them back to the nurses' home. As there was no place to talk privately (the sitting room was being used by others), Anne took them to her room. Soon afterwards, there was a knock on the door and the home warden demanded to know what was going on. Anne tried to explain, but was shouted down. Her sister also tried to speak and was similarly ignored. Angry, Anne, her sister and brother-in-law left the nurses' home and went to a nearby hotel for coffee.

The next day, Anne told several of her friends what had happened, and asked for their support at a meeting she intended to hold to get the rule on visiting changed. A week later, the first nurses' home meeting was held. The home warden, matron and other senior nurses were present. So were all the resident student nurses who were not on duty.

Anne explained that the meeting was being held to get a change in the rules about visitors to students in the home. It was not intended as a personal attack on the warden, but was aimed at drawing attention to the injustice of a blanket rule. At first, the warden was angry and accused Anne of breaking the rules and 'stirring up trouble', but it soon became clear that this was not the first time that an incident involving students' relatives had happened in the home. The students involved had grumbled, but did no more.

As leader of the meeting, Anne asked the warden to explain why the rule on visitors had been devised, and why it applied to relatives. The warden explained that there had been two or three pregnancies among the students; the rule had been established as a way of preventing further incidents, at least among resident nurses. She accepted that the rule should perhaps not apply to relatives, but argued that there was a need to keep the nurses in the home 'under control'.

Anne and the other students accepted that having male visitors in the home was risky, especially if the visitors wandered about unaccompanied (as they sometimes did). But what if the students were trusted to control themselves, and each other? After all, they were being asked to be in charge of wards full of sick people; surely they could be given the opportunity to show that they were more than capable of behaving responsibly? As it was, the rule was being broken regularly – at least one student had been censured for having her boyfriend living in her room at weekends. The other students had 'covered' for her, not because they believed she was right in what she was doing, but because they objected to the inflexibility of the rule. Other students said that Anne's outspokenness had been justified because everyone felt negatively about the rule. The matron agreed that the students should be trusted more, and that the rule would be reviewed. Anne suggested that it could still have 'teeth', and the students could get a better deal, if:

- all student nurses could have relatives visit them in their room, and would agree to inform the warden in advance
- students could have male friends visit them in the home twice weekly, in a designated room; the men would have to be escorted, and would not be left to wander around
- students would respect the fact that in an all-female home, some people would be alarmed at seeing unfamiliar men on the bedroom corridors
- if students had male friends stay overnight, they would be acting irresponsibly and unfairly in relation to their colleagues.

Everyone at the meeting agreed that these four initial changes would help in making the home a better place in which to live. Anne was pleased at the outcome of the meeting. She was not really prepared for the backlash.

For the next 3 months, Anne experienced increasing hostility from the warden. During that period she worked with a ward sister who was a personal friend of the warden. Anne was made to work every weekend over that 3 months (usually, students had alternate weekends off), and received a poor ward report at the end of her placement. Her boyfriend (also a student nurse) received similar treatment. Both were accused of telling lies against the warden, and of plotting to get the ward sister sacked. Such behaviour toward Anne continued, on and off, until the middle of her final year of training, when the ward sister retired. Anne completed her training successfully, and was later appointed to a senior staff nurse post at the hospital.

Talk to Anne today and she laughs about that time. She says she never set out to antagonize the warden, and was really scared that they would dismiss her and tell her mother (which was scarier!). 'I just wanted the unfairness to stop. Young people have always challenged unfairness and injustice. In my small way I was doing the same thing. I never thought they would turn nasty about it'.

Anne now knows she is a leader. But at the time of the home meeting, she just wanted to fix something that was not right. Looking back to when she was a child, Anne says that she was always the first to argue if something seemed wrong to her. 'My mother tells me that the first word I ever spoke clearly was 'Why!'. Today, Anne is still fighting to fix things that are not right. The goals are bigger, but her task as a leader is still the same – to challenge systems and change them.

A CRUEL PRACTICE – LISBETH MORGANAU

The central character in the next story is a midwife. She is shy, soft spoken, and wholly committed to making childbirth a positive and joyful experience for the women who come to her for care – women who, before her time in the hospital, trusted everything the doctors told them, and never questioned, never argued. In that hospital, a midwife or nurse challenging a doctor's orders was so rare as to be a novelty. But things change.

Lisbeth Morganau (not her real name) trained as a nurse and midwife in South Africa. She works in a hospital in the Transvaal, and likes being a midwife. A mix of women use the hospital services, and generally the care they receive is of high quality.

Lisbeth gets little time to pursue continuing education opportunities, but she reads professional journals and knows that midwifery practice in South Africa is not as advanced as in many other countries. Midwives there do not enjoy the same level of autonomy as, for instance, those in the UK.

Until recently, the country's healthcare system was heavily biased towards acute medicine, and doctors were prominent in all decisions about health care. With the ending of apartheid, primary care has moved to the centre of healthcare planning and delivery, but such large-scale changes tend to evolve slowly. In the meantime, midwives like Lisbeth Morganau have to work in the same environment as before, with the same people, and with the same problems.

One of those problems is the routine performance of episiotomies during delivery of first babies, regardless of size. Up until the early 1980s, many obstetricians demanded that all 'their primips' (first-time mothers) be given an episiotomy routinely. The rationale was to avoid damage to the woman's pelvic floor muscles from tears during delivery of the baby. Research, however, has proved that episiotomies (which are, after all, surgical interventions) can produce far worse morbidity for women than perineal tears. For example, the catgut sutures commonly used to repair episiotomies can cause poor healing, increased risk of infection, and allergic reaction. In response to such findings, sutures made from non-catgut material, which minimize the risk of infection and poor perineal healing, have been produced, and are now the first choice of many midwives and obstetricians worldwide.

Literature on such research was available in apartheid-era South Africa, but the journals in which research findings were published were frequently not accessible to nurses and midwives. Similarly, nurses and midwives were only very rarely allowed to attend international conferences where new knowledge and techniques would be described. It was therefore very difficult for midwives such as Lisbeth to keep up to date with developments.

Despite these handicaps, Lisbeth was aware that many first-time mothers suffered much pain following the routine performance of episiotomies, with infected wounds being common. She knew the women would not want them, given the choice. The midwives didn't want them either. They saw the distress, pain and illnesses they caused first-hand. But if they did not follow the doctors' instructions, they would find themselves in trouble, even if the woman laboured very quickly and no time was available to perform the procedure. If a woman suffered a perineal tear as a result, the midwife would be accused of negligence by the doctor. Even if, as was most commonly the case, the women suffered no tears, the doctors were still unhappy that their orders had not been carried out (at least Lisbeth did not work with doctors like the one heard about who, in one UK hospital which had a similar policy, performed an episiotomy on a first-time mother *after* delivery, to ensure the policy had been adhered to).

I met Lisbeth at a conference I attended in South Africa. She was a participant at a session at which I presented a paper. At the end of the session, Lisbeth approached me and told me her story about the routine episiotomies. She was clearly upset. During the session, some presenters had spoken about the positive developments in midwifery in their home countries. Lisbeth said that she felt that the women in her care were being short-changed, and that she felt powerless to challenge the doctors.

'How can I get it to change?', she asked. 'The doctors will not listen, and some of my colleagues will not support me in trying to change this'. Lisbeth wanted to know if there was any way that I could come and speak to her colleagues. That option not being a possibility at the time, we talked about past and current research from the UK on episiotomies – perineal tear versus episiotomy, the repair of episiotomies, and the prevention of perineal trauma during delivery.

Lisbeth was excited, but knew that the research papers alone would not necessarily convince the doctors in her hospital, or some of her midwife colleagues. She therefore decided that she would enlist help from her local university to set up small seminars to read and discuss the research, and compare the outcome of perineal tears and episiotomies for women having a first baby. She also wanted to start a network with midwives experiencing similar difficulties. When I left Lisbeth, she was busy talking with other midwives at the conference, asking about practices in their hospitals.

I cannot tell you how Lisbeth has fared. Whatever the outcomes, she has taken the first step to make the changes she wants to see. They may not all happen in her lifetime, but as South Africa re-integrates with the rest of the world, it will become easier for people like Lisbeth to challenge the status quo.

BABY LOVE – DR LYNDA RANDOLPH

I first heard about Lynda Randolph when I was organizing a 1-year research fellowship to the USA. Lynda, based in New York City, was suggested to me as someone who would be able to advise me on the best medical school to use as a base for the year, and who could help me to arrange the field work I needed to complete.

When I telephoned her to explore the options, I let it slip that I was also in need of a mentor for my time in the USA. Lynda asked if I would mind if she became my mentor. Ever an opportunist, I jumped. We had a few more telephone discussions, and arranged to meet on my first night in New York City. At that first meeting, she offered me sole use of her office at Mount Sinai Medical School while she was on secondment to the Carnegie Corporation. It was only after this that I realized that Lynda Randolph was way out of my league of leaders.

Lynda is a paediatrician and a specialist in maternal and child health. She has worked at the highest levels of government in New York State, including Director of Public Health at the State Health Department. An acknowledged authority on the development of children, she was the director of Project Head Start, a federally funded programme designed to enable children from disadvantaged areas to get a 'head start' in the educational system. During her time as director, Lynda opened Head Start to parents, especially women, as children's educational attainment is enhanced if their parents are also educated.

In addition to her demanding job, Lynda is also active in her local community. In the late 1970s, she was acutely aware of the disparity in neonatal mortality rates between white and black babies in New York City (1:1.7 deaths). This disparity was long-established, and had been a vexed political issue for some years. In the knowledge that poor or no access to health care during pregnancy is a major cause of premature deaths of minority ethnic babies in New York City, Lynda decided to work to change those statistics. She set up the New York City Perinatal Network, an association of community groups dedicated to improving the health of minority ethnic women and children. A decade later, there were three more perinatal networks serving Harlem, the Bronx, and Brooklyn.

Setting up the first network might seem to have been a gamble. After all, the USA in the 1970s and 1980s was not kind to poor people. There was growing resentment against those seen as 'feckless', and politicians were only too willing to grant the tax cuts demanded by those who believed the US welfare system had created whole cities of lazy, dependent, parasitic people. Lynda had a prestigious job in government, established academic credentials, and a bright future. Why mess all that up?

I made the error of asking just that question, in response to which Lynda laughed and said, 'Next question!' There has never been doubt in her mind that she owed her success and her prominent position to those who had earlier blazed the trail for minority ethnic people. Her contribution to maintaining that trail was to ensure that minority ethnic communities were healthy enough to produce others like her.

In the late 1980s a senior official in the administration of the then President, George Bush, reported that the health of babies in the USA was second worst in the world, after Bangladesh. As a result, in 1991, a 5-year programme, Healthy Start, was created, with the aim of reducing the neonatal mortality rate in minority communities by 50% by 1996. The Perinatal Networks initiated by Lynda became the centre of New York City's focus to achieve this aim.

People who now acknowledge the success of Healthy Start in New York City may know very little about Lynda Randolph. Like many high-achieving Americans, she has received numerous awards and citations, but in a one-to-one conversation, these are never mentioned. What she (passionately) agitates about is the worsening situation of many minority ethnic people, and the widening gap between those who can and those who cannot afford health care.

There is nothing pretentious or self-serving in this goal. Lynda, who has completed the executive management training programme at Harvard

Business School, argues the business as well as the compassionate case for affordable and accessible health care. She brings the same business-like attitude and compassion to leading people, taking tough decisions without causing loss of self-esteem (she has been know to fire people, and they leave her office laughing at one of her jokes). Like other effective leaders, Lynda does not hanker after recognition. She works to bring others together for a common purpose.

ONE MAN AND HIS MILL – AARON FEUERSTEIN (Teal 1996)

This story is straight out of a book. In fact, many people who know more than I do about these things argue that it cannot be out of a book – it is too unreal, if not unnatural. A business owner who, when disaster strikes, keeps on paying his staff, even though they are doing nothing? Here is the story. Judge for yourself.

Aaron Feuerstein is the owner, Chief Executive, and President of Malden Mills of Lawrence, Massachusetts. Malden Mills makes textiles. Its workers are probably the highest paid in the business, and the factory is based in the high-wage eastern seaboard area of the USA. It is a very successful company, more than tripling its revenues between 1982–1995, while barely doubling the number of employees. Ninety-five per cent of customers do repeat business with the company, and staff turnover is low, at less than five per cent.

Until the early 1980s, Malden Mills made its money by producing and selling artificial furs, but this market collapsed and alternative fabrics had to be found. The research and development and production staff at Malden Mills created a series of wool-like, thermal, resilient, lightweight fabrics, traded as Polartec and Polarfleece. These fabrics proved popular with people who like to exercise outdoors in cold weather, and have recently been used to make upholstery. All was now well at Malden Mills – that is, until the fire in 1996 which completely destroyed the Lawrence factory.

It is at this point that the opinions of business watchers and academics in the USA begin to differ. Aaron Feuerstein feels unappreciated, misunderstood and a little peeved that his instinctive response to the fire caused such extreme reactions. All he did was – continue to pay his staff while the factory was being re-built (a total of $15 million in wages and benefits), and re-build the factory in the same place.

For this act of what, in his eyes, is only supreme commonsense, Aaron Feuerstein has been called 'fool' by some, and 'saint' by others. He believes he is neither, because his decisions were simply based on very solid grounds:

• He believes that superior staff give superior service. Superior staff need to be rewarded appropriately, and superior service and products are not created by sweated labour.

- Malden Mills is a family firm. To have taken the insurance money and not re-build the factory would have meant billions of dollars of lost revenue to the family, as insurance companies pay out more for fire damage if funds are used to re-build a better factory.
- Unionized Malden Mills had a long tradition of replacing staff with new technology, but it had never had a strike and genuinely treated staff as its major asset.
- Staff had remained loyal to the company through the hard times in the 1980s. The expertise and experience of staff had been instrumental in Malden Mills' survival.
- While a devotee of downsizing (that is, reducing the size of the workforce), Feuerstein believes doing it for its own sake is a waste of valuable resources.
- He could not have moved the factory to a low wage state in the South of the USA, because wages in those states are rising.
- Moving the business to a country like Thailand would have lost Malden Mills the irreplaceable advantage of being a producer of the highest quality goods, for the temporary advantage of low wages.

There are those who believe Feuerstein has been touched by God, and those who believe he is simply touched. But in truth, he was just practising what he had preached for decades. All said, Feuerstein's story is a near-textbook example of consistent leadership. He was not seeking recognition when he made his decision; he was doing what effective leaders always do – setting an example for others to follow.

ONLY A PLEB – ALISON MENNIE

It started with a cup of coffee and an article in a magazine.

Since qualifying 10 years ago, Alison Mennie has worked in oncology, a speciality to which she had been attracted since her first year of training. While working in Cambridge on a radiology unit, Alison noticed that mouth care for patients having chemotherapy was not satisfactory. Shortly after, she left the UK for Canada, where she worked in a bone marrow transplant unit for 2 years. On her return to the UK, she was unable to get a job on a similar unit, and opted to work as an agency nurse.

One of her placements was at the St. John's Hospice in Doncaster, where the matron was the first person ever to show interest in Alison's stint in Canada. Alison joined the hospice's nurse bank, which led to a temporary, 1-year contract. To increase her expertise and knowledge, she completed ENB 931 – Continuing Care of the Dying Patient and the Family. She was then appointed on a longterm contract at St. John's.

Alison's concerns about the efficacy of mouth care for dying people had never subsided. Wherever she went in the UK or Canada, there was no method of mouth care that was satisfactory to the patient or to her. Like all leaders who find a problem, Alison wanted to solve it. She started doing the research on mouth care – which is where the article comes in.

One morning, Alison was having coffee and reading a magazine, when she spotted an article on Tea Tree Oil. She was struck by the many uses of this product, including the fact that Tea Tree Oil is a powerful anti-fungal agent. The fungal infection of oral thrush is a common complaint for people who have had chemotherapy. Alison made the connection: why not use Tea Tree as a mouth care agent?

Thrush and other fungal mouth infections cause pain. This leads to difficulties in eating, talking, and sleeping. Difficulties in sleeping causes irritability, and a reluctance to take part in activities of any kind. An apparently simple mouth infection can therefore have serious consequences. Alison wrote to the matron, set out her thoughts, and asked to conduct a study to test the effectiveness of Tea Tree Oil as a mouth care agent. Using her own money to buy the oil, Alison began her study (using as a framework, the Scope of Professional Practice), after she had first tried the product on herself.

Alison talked to her colleagues about the study. They were interested, but sceptical. They became convinced, however, after the results with the first patient were presented: the solution of two drops of oil to 100 millilitres of water, first applied with a spongette, then used as a mouth wash, had removed every trace of white plaque from the patient's mouth. The patient was overjoyed, and comfortable for the first time in months. Alison was astonished. Subsequently, all the patients in the study received great relief from using the oil for mouth care. They ate, slept, and generally felt better.

Since Alison's study, only one patient has been prescribed conventional anti-fungal agents for mouth infections in 2 years. The oil has been adopted by an aromatherapist to produce air fresheners for rooms in the hospice and, in one case, to deodorize dressing pads. The oil is now regularly supplied through pharmacy, and Alison's colleagues, nurses and doctors, are no longer sceptical.

I first read about Alison's work from her application to the 1997 *Nursing Times* / 3M Awards, of which I was a judge. She had seen an advertisement for the Award on a wall in the hospice, and applied. Alison was one of five first-place winners of the Award. On receiving her prize from the Secretary of State for Health, I overheard her say, 'I am only a pleb'. Yet the behaviour, aptitude, and mind-set of this leader is anything but plebian.

What Alison Mennie's work with Tea Tree Oil has proved is that the best kind of nursing care comes from putting the patient at the centre of our thinking. Alison also demonstrates another attribute of leadership which I will discuss in Chapter 5 – leaders focus on solutions, not problems.

COULD IT BE YOU?

You have probably read these stories with gritted teeth. The problem with stories about leaders is that they seem perfect – obstacles surmounted, disaster averted, round of applause. They make it look so easy. They do not have crumbling hospitals to deal with, or truly awful managers to work for. They seem to have endless imagination, and friends in all the right places. Seem to.

Probably all of the people whose stories I have just shared with you would agree that what they have accomplished is worthy of note. But that is after the event. When you set out to do something, it rarely crosses your mind that the result might create a marker for others to follow. You just feel the urgent need to change something, find the solution to a problem, help others achieve an objective, or finish what has already been started. This may be the only part of the theories about leadership that do not start to crumble when touched by reality.

Let me set the context of the next two chapters, which deal with the reality of leadership in health care and the characteristics that mark out effective and successful leaders respectively, by highlighting some issues about the people in the stories above.

None of these people was born to be a leader. They do not fit the 'Great Man' theory referred to in Chapter 3, but they do fit the model of situational leadership. Remember that this type of leader works out the particular and general needs of a given set of circumstances, and then chooses an approach which is appropriate. She or he will then monitor how effective they have been. All of the people above share many of the characteristics of this style – they are creative, credible, willing to challenge the status quo, take risks, share power, and be versatile. Situational leaders make themselves, or are made. They are not born as leaders. None of us is.

The people in the stories above also exhibit those qualities which draw people – warmth, approachability, strong people-focus, emotional stability, and consistency (that is, living and acting by a set of principles). Aaron Feuerstein's act of keeping all his staff on the pay-roll while the factory was rebuilt, for example, is the outcome of his belief that caring about employees, quality service, and customers are not incompatible goals. He simply practised what he preached.

Anne Smith could not have named one theory of leadership, but she knew that there had to be a better way to treat nurses who lived in the nurses' home. Lynda Randolph knows a great deal about leadership theories, yet her approach was to work through community, not formal, organizational structures. Mary Seacole and Lisbeth Morganau challenged the establishment in the form of government and doctors, and did it on their own. Alison Mennie had long felt nurses 'could do better' for patients who had special mouth care needs.

For every leader who comes to public notice, there are several hundred others who, lights burning steadily behind bushels, get on with the job. You already know what type of leader inspires you, and you may have begun to model yourself on this person. But modelling does not mean losing heart if you do not achieve as much as they did. You have to write your own stories (and tell them), dream your own dreams, and learn to be the best leader you can be.

Key learning points

- Leaders are persistent in their approach to achieving their goals.

- Few leaders take 'no' for an answer.

- Leaders give in, but never give up.

- Sometimes you have to go it alone to achieve an objective.

- Leadership and authority are not necessarily the same thing.

- Leaders are made, not born.

REFERENCES

Alexander Z, Dewjee A 1984 The wonderful adventures of Mrs Seacole in many lands, 2nd edn. Falling Water Press, Bristol
Audit Commission 1997 Finders keepers: the management of staff turnover in NHS Trusts. Audit Commission, London
De Pree M 1989 Leadership is an art. Arrow, London
Kouzes J M, Posner B Z 1987 The leadership challenge: how to get extraordinary things done in organizations. Jossey-Bass, San Francisco
Kouzes J M, Posner B Z 1995 The leadership challenge: how to keep getting extraordinary things done in organizations. Jossey-Bass, San Francisco
Moss Kanter R 1977 Men and women of the corporation. Basic Books, New York
Peters T, Waterman R 1995 In search of excellence. HarperCollins, London
Teal T 1996 Not a fool, not a saint. Fortune, 11 November: 111–113

Theorizing about leaders and leadership

Key words:

organization theory; situational leadership; contingency leadership; transactional and transformational leadership; different ways of leading

It is possible to talk about theories of leadership without considering the social, cultural, and organizational structures within which leaders operate, but this would be artificial. In the first part of this chapter, we will take a very quick trip around the outskirts of organization theory, making a detour to peer at the socio-cultural frameworks which influence ideas about leaders and leadership. We can then given our attention to the vast literature on leadership, with a focus on the 20th century (or we will never end). At the end of the chapter is a list of books which cover many aspects of organization theory and leadership theory. Most are easy to find and easy to read, and I will be referring to some of them by name.

THEORIES OF ORGANIZATIONS

By organization theory, I mean the ideas that exist about how organizations are designed and managed, their function, cultures and operations, and how people within them are rewarded and motivated. For simplicity, organization theory can be classified into 'schools' of thought:

- The Classic School (focus: organization structure and function)
- The Human Relations School (focus: people in organizations and how they make sense of work)

- The Marxist School (focus: how capitalism, in organizational form, exploits workers).

The Classic School

The main proponents are a Scot, Frederick Taylor, and his school of scientific management, and Henri Fayol (a Frenchman). Both were engineers. Taylor believed that 'the principle object of management should be to secure the maximum prosperity for the employer, coupled with maximum prosperity of the employee' (Pugh & Hickson 1989). To achieve this, four things had to happen:

1. Employers had to know exactly what constituted a fair day's work.
2. Workers had to be scientifically selected to ensure that they had the intellectual and physical capacity to deliver the required performance.
3. Managers needed to manage according to scientific methods.
4. There had to be 'constant and intimate' cooperation between workers and managers.

Taylor was criticized in his lifetime for the apparent inhumanity of his system. With its emphasis on efficiency, many people felt that Taylor viewed workers as little more than well-oiled machines. An attempt to implement his ideas in a US government arsenal provoked a workers' strike and led the US House of Representatives into calling a special hearing to investigate his methods.

In truth, however, Taylor was also very critical of managers' failure to get the best from workers. He advocated that the earnings of workers who produced the most should not be limited, yet every incentive scheme devised since then to increase productivity and reward good performance has been capped. Remember performance related pay?

Fayol formulated similar ideas to Taylor's. He provided a definition of management which is still relevant today. Paraphrasing his 'five elements' of management, Fayol claimed that to manage is to:

1. forecast and plan
2. organize
3. command (that is, ensure that the tasks get done)
4. coordinate
5. control.

These five elements have helped clear the mind of many managers, especially those struggling in their first substantive managerial role. Fayol also devised 14 General Principles of Management, which included equity ('a combination of kindliness and justice is needed to ensure that everyone receives equal treatment'), and unity of command ('each employee must have one boss') (Pugh & Hickson 1989). How evident have these been in the NHS recently?

Taylor, Fayol and others with similar ideas still influence how organizations are structured, how they function and how the people who work in them are rewarded. Call centres, for instance, operate on Taylorite lines. Traces of Taylor are also visible in National Vocational Qualifications (NVQs), management competencies, and management by objectives. Fayol's definition of management has survived nearly 50 years of vigorous debate and arguments, and his 14 Principles are still clearly visible in most organizations.

The Human Relations School

In a nutshell, the Human Relations (or Behavioural) School of management holds that people work better when they are involved in decisions about their work, and are treated as human beings. The person most often associated with these ideas is Elton Mayo, an Australian who spent most of his working life at Harvard University. Mayo is also credited with being the founder of industrial sociology, or the study of how people behave at work.

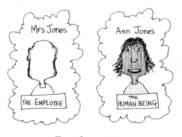

People matter

From 1927 to 1932, Mayo and a group of like-minded associates investigated worker productivity at the Hawthorne factory of the Western Electric Company in Chicago. These research projects have become known throughout the world as 'The Hawthorne Experiments'.

Their task was to find out why there were variances in worker performance. In the first part of the investigation, Mayo and his team studied the output of six women who assembled telephone equipment. The women were removed from their usual 48-hour, 6-day week and were subjected to various changes – a special payment scheme, shorter hours, refreshments, and rest periods of varying lengths. The study tested the impact of these changes on morale and performance, before the women were returned to their normal work routine. At each change, the women were involved in the planning and execution of the phase (Mayo 1933).

During the 5 years the women were involved in the experiment, performance and morale improved, incentives or not. Mayo concluded that the specific changes had not been responsible for the production increase, and he was unable to explain at the time what had caused the improvements. Later, he suggested that feeling important and valued were more important to people than having good physical conditions of work. In other words, fine new buildings are no substitute for effective group dynamics.

A key finding of Mayo's work was that employees and managers had different perspectives – employees were driven by what he called the 'logic of sentiment', while managers were more concerned with the 'logic of cost and efficiency'. If both sides can understand their different 'switch points', Mayo argued, destructive conflict can be avoided. The key is mutual respect and communication.

The lasting significance of the Hawthorne Experiments was the confirmation of the existence of the informal organization, the 'virtual' place that gives the formal organization its stability through the formation of social relationships. Mayo also disproved the still commonly held view that workers are propelled by narrow self-interest. In Mayo's view, the role of managers was to create the conditions in which 'spontaneous cooperation' and group affiliation can flourish, while maintaining the 'logic of cost and efficiency'. 'Management', he wrote, 'succeeds or fails in proportion as it is accepted without reservation by the group as authority and leader'.

The Marxist School

Marxists are scathing of both the Classic and the Human Relations schools – the Classicals because their ideas are manipulated to give capitalists control over workers, and Human Relationists who, Marxists believe, want to humanize a fundamentally debased system of work.

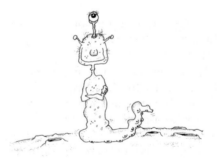

Ai(ling) (lien-a)

The leading Marxist theorist on organizations was Harry Braverman (Braverman 1974). He was particularly dismissive of the Human Relations

School whose ideas, he argued, are shunted to the sidelines of every organization, while Taylorism reigns at every level. In the end, according to his theories, all workers are de-skilled, society is just one huge marketplace, and the degradation of social and family life is the inevitable consequence.

Given the sameness of products in the shops and television programmes, and the vertical integration of business (overlapping ownership of newspapers, football clubs, television stations, etc.), Braverman's views seem to be spot-on. But it is not only managers who strive to exert control – company owners, employees and professional groups all fight to protect their interests. Contrary to Braverman's expectation that de-skilled white collar workers would join the working class, we now know that downsized, de-skilled managers tend to consider themselves to be middle-class, and have political views to match.

Take a moment now to consider your own organization through the following questions:

- Does it have Taylorite tendencies?
- Is there evidence of the 'spontaneous cooperation' that Mayo described?
- What do you think of Braverman's argument that the ideas of Mayo and others in the Human Relations School do not have centre-stage in an organization?
- Is nursing more Taylor than Mayo?
- Does any of this matter?

Let us move on.

LEADER TYPES

Notions of leadership are wrapped up with ideas of how organizations function. They also reflect the times in which they are formulated. Later (Chapter 9) we will talk about the influence of social norms on research on leadership. For now, I want to introduce you to the leader types you are most likely to meet on your journey to increase your effectiveness as a leader. I will try to give relevant examples of each type, either by name or by behaviour. As we progress, see how many real-life examples you can spot.

A quick summary of the types:

- The Great Man (or born to lead)
- The situational/contingency leader
- The transactional leader, and the transformational leader
- The non-corporate leader
- The relationship-based leader (Leader–Member Exchange, LMX Theory).

Later on, we will look in more detail at two of these types – the transformational leader, and the non-corporate leader.

The Great Man (or born to lead)

The era when the Great Man (or Trait Approach) theory of leadership was most closely studied was (roughly) 1930–1950. The focus of the theory was the person of the leader, the notion that a certain type of person was a leader for all seasons. Factors such as intellect, personality, height, class and age were investigated to find an identikit formula. Researchers were looking for the secret ingredient of leadership success.

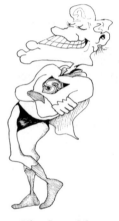

The Great Man

While some seekers identified precise features (6′2″, white, male, educated at Harvard, upper class, extrovert, etc.), others were less successful in their search. But the Great Man still persists in the imagination, in the form of a Hero. He is to be found in the pages of many (mainly US) business magazines, the business section of newspapers, in the autobiography section of any good book seller, and in the job pages ('Wanted – a born leader. Must have superior intellect, be outgoing, and under 40. Ability to walk on water a distinct advantage'). Unfortunately, they are also well represented in Chapter 8 of this book – Why Leaders Fail.

The Great Man theory persists because we, the people, are still searching for Him.

The situational/contingency leader

Having failed to identify the definitive Great Man, researchers sensibly turned their attention away from leaders' personality traits to concentrate on how they behaved. For the next 20 years, to the mid 1970s, several researchers focused on this area. It is fair to say that the seeds of much of what we know about leadership today, including transformational leadership, were sown and scattered during this period.

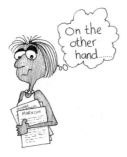

Several scholars (predominantly American) led the field, with Fred Fiedler, Rensis Likert, Douglas McGregor, and Tannenbaum and Schmidt prominent. I want to focus on Tannenbaum and Schmidt, and on the work of Fred Fiedler.

In 1958, the Harvard Business Review published an article by Tannenbaum and Schmidt entitled *How to Choose a Leadership Pattern* (Tannenbaum & Schmidt 1958). This article, now a classic, drew a clear distinction between managers who make decisions using their position and authority in an organization (autocrats), and those who have a more participative style (democrats). Tannenbaum and Schmidt proposed that leaders operate along a style spectrum – from 'boss-centered' autocrat, to 'subordinate-centered' democrat. The closer the leader was to being an autocrat, the less freedom subordinates had to be involved in decision-making; the closer to democrat, the more freedom for subordinates (see Fig. 3.1).

This theory became the framework for later research and management development initiatives, but cumulative data showed that while a participative management style produced more job satisfaction for subordinates, it did not necessarily produce a concomitant improvement in performance. The participative style was not effective in ensuring the successful completion of those routine tasks in which efficiency and time were key elements. Further research revealed that when these two seemingly independent aspects of leadership behaviour – concern for people or relationships, and concern for completion of tasks – appeared in the same person, a new style of leader emerged – the situational/contingency leader.

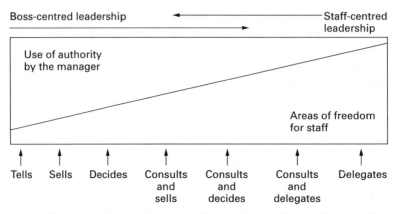

Figure 3.1 Continuum of leadership (adapted by permission of Harvard Business Review from Tannenbaum and Schmidt 1958. How to choose a leadership pattern. Harvard Business Review 36(2): 95–101. Copyright © 1958 by the President and Fellows of Harvard College, all rights reserved).

There are many models of this style of leadership, but one of the most influential is that set out in Fred Fielder's book, *A Theory of Leadership Effectiveness*. (Fiedler 1967). Fiedler argued that effective leadership is contingent on the job to be done, and the situations in which the leader has to operate. He developed a measure to classify the two leadership styles he described (relationship motivated, and task motivated). His arguments can be difficult to grasp, but his theory of contingency leadership has added immeasurably to our understanding of leadership. It also stands in complete contrast to the Great Man theory.

Much of Feidler's work sought to analyze how the leader can wield power and influence within the work group, and manage to retain respect and affection. He argued that the leader had to be aware of and sensitive to the dynamics in three particular dimensions of leadership:

1. The relationship between the leader and group members. The more mutual respect and liking, the more influence the leader would have in the group. Fiedler stressed that this is the single most important influence on leadership.
2. The leader's position power. Leaders who were able to reward and punish had more power and control than those who could not.
3. The tasks to be accomplished. Working with clear, specific tasks gave the leader more influence than when tasks were ambiguous or unstructured.

Another interesting part of his work involved asking leaders in the study to think of all the people they had worked with, and choose the one with whom they worked least well. They were then asked to rate this person (called the 'least preferred co-worker', or LPC) using a number of characteristics. Fielder found that:

- Leaders who were more relationship-motivated scored the characteristics highly no matter what the difficulties with LPC. For example, the LPC might be rated as lazy and inconsiderate, but warm. This type of leader was so concerned to maintain relationships that she or he would strive to discriminate fairly.
- Task-motivated leaders were focused on how people contributed to getting the job done. So the LPC would not only be lazy and inconsiderate, but also boring and miserable.

Fiedler emphasized that both these styles could be effective, if used in the appropriate circumstances. Although contingency and situational theories of leadership were once viewed separately, it is now generally accepted that they both focus on the same issue – the search for the most important elements in determining leadership style. The emphasis, therefore, is on competency, and the task is to discover a range of skills that are potentially teachable. Whether or not you agree with this premise, it is surely an improvement on the idea that leaders are born, not made, and that only certain types of personalities can aspire to such Olympian heights!

The transactional leader and the transformational leader

Both the Great Man theory and contingency/situational theories assumed an authority relationship between the leader and the follower. But as research developed, a paradigm shift occurred in thinking about leadership.

Remember that ideas about leadership reflect what is happening in a given society at a given time; social, technological and economic changes impact on how leaders and leadership are perceived. Great Man and contingency/situational theories were developed in a relatively predictable, stable world with comparative economic certainty. But the major recession of the 1980s, which affected most world economies, caused organizations to revise their operating methods and structures. This was the beginning of 'downsizing' and 'rightsizing', as large centrally-controlled organizations sought ways to respond to rapidly changing social, technological and economic environments.

'Top-down', militaristic forms of management were no longer appropriate. This new, fast-moving, and unstable world needed a new kind of leader, one who could help an organization successfully adapt to change. Writers and researchers on leadership became less interested in how leaders behaved, and focused more on what their followers said they wanted in a leader. The old leadership styles were now referred to as 'transactional' (or management), the new ones as 'transformational'.

The terms 'transactional leadership' and 'transformational leadership' were first used by Douglas McGregor Burns in 1978 (McGregor Burns 1978), and were later developed by two groups of US researchers working independently – Bernard Bass and Bruce Avolio, and James Kouzes and Barry Posner. We will look at transformational leadership in detail in Chapters 9 and 10, but an outline of the concept is necessary to illustrate the radical re-thinking about leadership that began in the mid-1980s.

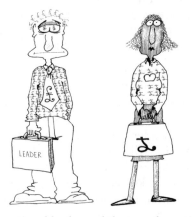

The transactional leader and the transformational leader

In two major and independent studies, Bass and Avolio, and Kouzes and Posner formulated models of transformational leadership based on analyses of how managers described their leadership experiences. Bass and Avolio's model identified four components of transformational leadership, called the 'Four Is' (Bass & Avolio 1994):

1. Leaders who are *individually considerate* treat their followers according to their needs. Assignments are delegated to provide learning and development opportunities.
2. The *intellectually stimulating leader* encourages people to challenge current ways of working, and to be creative. Questioning values, beliefs and expectations (individual as well as the organization's) is positively supported.
3. Charismatic leaders (or '*idealized influence*') are role models for their followers, who identify with their vision. These leaders are respected, trusted, have high standards and referent power (that is, they are power symbols). They help followers to overcome obstacles.
4. *Inspirational leaders* create optimism, and bring an emotional element to the work to be done (for example, appealing to people's desire to be 'part of something special'). While some elements may be similar to those of charismatic leaders, followers may not choose to emulate such a leader.

This research provided the stimulus for Kouzes and Posner's model. In their first study in 1987 (Koujes & Posner 1987), they asked 5000 managers to share their 'personal best' experiences as leaders. From the analysis of responses, they identified what they have called the 'five fundamentals of exemplary leadership'. While having similarities with Bass and Avolio's model, Kouzes and Posner's fundamentals highlight much more specific leadership behaviour (Box 3.1).

Box 3.1   Kouzes and Posner's fundamentals of exemplary leadership (adapted from Alimo-Metcalfe 1996)

Inspiring a shared vision
Leaders create a vision of the future. They have a desire to do things differently and inspire others by articulating a common purpose, and by finding out what their hopes and dreams are.

Modelling the way
Leaders act with integrity, setting an example by doing what they say they will do. They never expect others to do what they would not do. They also plan and review work in progress, and take corrective action as necessary.

Challenging the process
Experimentation, new ideas, devolved decision-making, and innovation as encouraged by leaders. They are therefore willing to take calculated risks. Leaders support followers when they make mistakes, which they view as part of learning.

Encouraging the heart
Achieving any vision is tiring, and can be frustrating. Leaders maintain morale by celebrating successes, recognizing achievement, and by visibly valuing their followers. Their praise is sincere, and they expect that their staff will always perform well.

Enabling others to act
Leaders enlist the support of others to achieve their vision. They work collaboratively and in partnerships, building effective working relationships with customers, staff, peers, and suppliers. Leaders also build strong teams, and use delegation as a method of staff development.

The models of leadership described by Bass and Avolio and Kouzes and Posner view followers as the constituents of leaders and not, as was previously the case, as passive onlookers. Leaders following the models commit to enabling themselves and their followers to optimize skills, abilities, knowledge and potential, and encourage innovation and challenges to how the organization does its business.

This sounds very exciting, and it is rare to hear an organization leader these days say anything other than 'our staff are our greatest asset'. But the reality in many organizations is that staff who follow the status quo are rewarded, while those who are critical, have innovative ideas, and are independent thinkers are soon off the premises. Writers on leadership emphasize that organizations require both transformational and transactional leaders. Kotter argues that leaders who cannot manage, and managers who cannot lead, give us the worst of both worlds (Kotter 1990). For many thousands of employees in many thousands of organizations, the worst of both worlds is a daily fact of life.

So, what can be done to help organizations' chief executives to practise what they preach, and begin to work on transformational lines? Can transformational leadership skills be learned? Researchers and writers are split on this. One of the problems is being able to scientifically define and measure what transformational leadership 'is'. Transactional leadership (or management) consists of a range of competencies which can be identified and measured – planning, controlling, problem-solving, productivity levels. Transformational leadership is more about attitudes and qualities which are not easily measured – showing respect for others, valuing different opinions, encouraging innovation and criticism, and possessing high levels of optimism. It might make sense to suggest, therefore, that transformational leadership is more dependent on innate features of the individual, rather than being something she or he can be taught.

Writers such as Abraham Zaleznik believe that individuals are either 'managers' or 'leaders', and that each has very different outlooks on the world (Alimo-Metcalfe 1996). Where managers relate to roles and act to limit choices, leaders take risks, are more concerned with ideas, and are more intuitive and empathetic. Bass believes that individuals who have a predominantly transactional style have more difficulty becoming transformational. But there is growing evidence from US studies that giving managers feedback on their performance, and following up with activities such as coaching and mentoring can result in a change in behaviour. We know that people can be socialized into holding certain attitudes early in life – why not later in life as well? Perhaps old dogs *can* be taught new tricks.

Judy Rosener's work has added another dimension to our understanding of transformational leadership – that of gender. In an article in the November/December 1990 issue of the Harvard Business Review called *Ways Women Lead* (Rosener 1990), Rosener described a survey which investigated men and women leaders. The results indicated that there were fundamental differences in how women and men described leadership. Briefly, men were more likely to describe themselves in terms that characterized transactional leadership; women were more likely to take a transformational approach to leadership.

As is the case with many pioneering studies, Rosener's work was greeted with scepticism. It was claimed that the results were unreliable because they were based on self-reports, and that no other researcher had found such differences (hardly surprising, given that until the mid-1980s, most of the research on leadership had focused on men; when women were included, it was to measure them against the male norm). But Rosener had simply asked different questions, and received different answers.

Using the now respected Multi-factor Leadership Questionnaire (MLQ),

Bass and Avolio followed up Rosener's work with a survey involving the followers of hundreds of female and male managers. Rosener's results were confirmed. We will look at the implications of this landmark study later in the book.

Nearly all of the research on transformational leadership has emanated from the USA, and has been based on the private commercial sector. UK research in this aspect of leadership is still in its infancy, but important work is now being carried out. For instance, the Local Government Board commissioned a research project on transformational leadership in local government, and a similar survey in the NHS was sponsored by the Nuffield Institute for Health in Leeds. Both surveys were conducted by Professor Beverly Alimo-Metcalfe, who used some of the items from Bass and Avolio's MLQ, and concentrated on issues such as political skills, self-awareness/humility, intellectual capacity and time management, in addition to all of Bass and Avolio's Four Is'. These surveys were less gender-biased than the US studies, and this may in part account for the greater complexity of the model of transformational leadership that emerged from the studies (Alimo-Metcalfe 1996).

Several conclusions were drawn:

- The UK model of transformational leadership which emerged from the surveys is very different from the US one.
- The most important factors associated with transformational leadership are different in the two countries – in the USA it is charisma, in the UK it is empathy and actively supporting the individual's development. Both sets of factors are present in US and UK studies, but in different orders of importance.
- The factors 'intellectual capacity', and 'self-awareness/humility' (willing to admit mistakes or say 'I don't know') do not emerge from US surveys.
- There are specific dimensions in the UK survey which reflect the political environment of local government and the NHS, such as political skills, credibility with various stakeholders, and working with elected officials.

The UK as a whole have yet to take leadership issues seriously. Most UK organizations, including those in the public sector, are increasingly obsessed with competencies (for example the Management Charter Initiative, and NVQs), which reflect transactional leadership. The maxim 'what gets measured, gets done' emphasizes management, with its focus on order, adaptation, certainty and stability. The reality of organizational life, however, is rapid and increasing change, which demands flexibility, judicious risk-taking, innovation, and development of individuals' potential. Transformational leadership may be complex, not easily measurable (if at all) and potentially frustrating, but the alternative is to continue to depend on the transactional leadership style, which is not amenable to enabling and sustaining change and organizational survival.

The non-corporate leader

So far, we have looked at leadership in the formal context of organizations, largely because that has been the focus of writers and researchers on leadership. I believe that this approach has had the unfortunate effect of limiting our perspective on leadership, and has left the impression that leadership is an activity that takes place within the confines of work relationships. But the concept of leadership has no boundaries. We know that it does not reside in one type of person, nor is it limited to one gender, race, class, or nationality. It is a truly universal idea, and as such is subject to social, economic, and technological influences. Yet almost nothing is known about how leadership manifests outside formal organizations, in the environment where there are numerous examples of its forms – local communities.

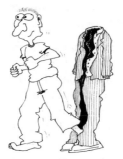

The non-corporate leader

My interest in what I call 'non-corporate forms of leadership' dates from the late 1970s, and the birth of self-help movements which focused on health (especially women's health). I was particularly fascinated by the response of the health and social service sector to involving service users in planning and delivering services. As a midwife, I saw evidence of this in my daily practice, which was heavily influenced by the growing demands of pregnant women and their supporters for more humane maternity services and less medical intervention during pregnancy and childbirth.

More than a decade later, researching and studying models of community involvement sharpened my interest. Part of this research took place in New York City, where I was attached to the Brooklyn Perinatal Network (BPN) in the Bedford-Stuyvesant area of Brooklyn. The project had grown out of 20 years of the community taking the lead to improve education, policing, health, street cleaning, the environment, and any other factor which they perceived as not enhancing their community. A few people, from different parts of the community and with very different backgrounds and interests, decided to make a difference.

It was particularly fascinating to observe the local people take on the mantle of negotiating with the paid professionals (health officials, politicians, etc). One afternoon, I attended one of the regular meetings between the staff and board of BPN, also attended by officials from the federal and state government, to discuss progress on a major project aimed at reducing infant mortality in the area. I noticed differences in the way the various parties spoke about the project concerned. Community activists/leaders on the board spoke with an absence of cant, but with passion and street savvy, and were very focused on outcomes; the officials, and those board members who were professional healthcare workers or administrators, spoke the language of organizational rhetoric – measurement, outputs, the need for caution, minimum data sets, financial accountability. Community activists/leaders addressed racialism as a key issue underlying the need for the project; the officials never once gave attention to race, even though the focus of the project was infant mortality which, as we have seen in Chapter 2, affects more black than white babies in the USA.

Bedford-Stuyvesant is the last place that you might expect to find leaders and leadership. The area has a woeful history of deprivation, racialism and general neglect by local and state government. But leaders will emerge in the places where change is needed, and change was certainly needed in Bedford-Stuyvesant. The BPN project and other examples of non-corporate leadership models are discussed in much detail later, but if you cannot wait, then turn to Chapter 12 now.

Box 3.2 Some characteristics of non-corporate settings

- No normal structures, or formal leaders.
- Proceedings are more fluid, and random.
- Less formality among participants.
- Leaders emerge out of events.
- Leaders depend more on personal power (influence) than on resource and position power.
- Leaders may only lead with the consent of the group.
- Leadership role changes hands on several occasions.
- Confusion, factionalism, and divided loyalties.

Box 3.2 gives a summary of the characteristics of non-corporate settings and the type of leadership role produced. Suffice to say that I have observed more transformational than transactional tendencies (although I am sure that there are exceptions to this).

The relationship-based leader (Leader–Member Exchange or LMX theory)

The focus of these leaders is the relationship they form with each member of their team or group. Central to this relationship is the quality of communications between the leader and the group.

In a nutshell, each group tends to consists of two sub-groups – the in-group and the out-group. Both groups work differently, which in turn affects the way they work with, relate to and communicate with the leader.

The in-group are concerned to expand their roles beyond the job description and actively negotiate with the leader to make this happen. In turn, the leader does more with (and for) this group, who receive more information, more communication, and generally have more connections within the wider organization. The in-group are also more personally compatible with the leaders.

Conversely, the out-group are more focused on self-interest, the formal employment contract and limits of the prescribed job in hand. They are not interested in expanding their role, and are less compatible with the leader. Members of this group come to work, do their job, and go home.

Sounds familiar? You might be able to work out the in-groups and out-groups in your own organization, and define where you stand. But part of the leader's job is to ensure the these groups do not form in the first place. It is a natural instinct for us to want to work mostly with those people we like, or who are similar to us in some way. This instinct is no less strong for leaders, because remember – leaders R us. To be effective, however, leaders must build successful relationships with *all* the members of the group, finding ways to accommodate the varying levels of interest, commitment, and energy found in every group.

The presence of in- and out-groups can become divisive, leading to accusations of favouritism being levelled at the leader. Research on LMX theory suggests that high quality relationships between the leader and the *whole* group leads to lower levels of staff turn-over, better job appraisals, more commitment, and greater participation. The organization benefits by being more productive, and more successful (Northouse 1997). LMX theory emphasizes the importance of 'leadership-making' – the need for leaders to build effective relationships with a variety of people. The three phases of leadership-making are summarized in the Box 3.3.

WHAT NEXT?

The UK lags behind the USA in terms of research on leadership but it is catching up. This is not surprising, because the current emphasis on 'management' rather than 'leadership' in organizations such as the NHS is causing big problems. While chief executives neglect their assigned leadership

---

Box 3.3 The phases of leadership-making (adapted from Northouse 1997)

1. *The Stranger* – the relationship is bound by rules, contracts, prescribed roles, hierarchy. The quality of communications is limited to the immediate task in hand and the quality may be poor.
2. *The Acquaintance* – the relationship begins to include social exchanges, more sharing of information (both work-related and personal), more trust. Each party (leader and group member) is 'testing the water', the leader to see how ready the group member is to take on new challenges, the group member to consider if the challenges are worthwhile. The quality of communication improves as mutual respect increases.
3. *The Partner* – the relationship is characterized by trust, mutual respect, and mutual feelings of obligation. This is a mature relationship where interdependence is accepted, there is a high level of reciprocity, and exchange of favours. Each partner has developed very effective ways of communicating and relating, which produces many positive benefits for them and the organization. In essence, they have a transformational relationship.

---

role, staff revolt with their feet. Those who do choose to lead are largely unsupported, and many take their passion elsewhere. People-intensive services like the NHS need to take an active interest in theories of leadership, and of organizations. One consequence of not doing so is to continue to make the same mistakes in the same way, with the same unhappy results.

Key learning points

- Ideas about leadership are influenced by social, technological, and economic changes.

- Frederick Taylor is alive and well, and living it up in many organizations (including the NHS).

- The Great Man theory of leadership is still alive in some people's minds.

- There are fundamental differences between the UK and US models of transformational leadership.

- Not all leaders are found inside formal organizations.

- Leaders can be made.

REFERENCES

Alimo-Metcalfe B 1996 Leaders or managers? Nursing Management 3(1): 22–24
Bass B M, Avolio B J 1994 Shatter the glass ceiling: women may make better managers. Human Resource Management 33(4): 549–560

Braverman H 1974 Labour – monopoly capitalism: the segregation of work in the twentieth century. Monthly Review Press, New York

Fayol H 1949 General and industrial management. IEEE Publications, Middlesex

Fiedler F 1967 A theory of leadership effectiveness. McGraw-Hill, New York

Kotter J 1990 A force for change: how leadership differs from management. Free Press, London

Kouzes J, Posner B 1987 The leadership challenge: how to get extraordinary things done in organizations. Jossey-Bass, San Francisco

McGregor Burns J 1978 Leadership. HarperCollins, New York

Mayo E 1933 The human problems of an industrial civilisation. Macmillan, London

Northouse P G 1997 Leadership – theory and practice. Sage Publications, London

Pugh D S, Hickson D J 1989 Writers on organizations. Penguin, London

Rosener J B 1990 Ways women lead. Harvard Business Review 68(6): 119–125

Tannenbaum R, Schmidt W H 1958 How to choose a leadership pattern. Harvard Business Review 36(2): 95–101

4

Theory and practice

Key words:

reality; ethics and emotion; support; nurses as leaders; *Star Trek*; language

Personal experience tells me that theories about leadership and organizations are put into practice very sparingly in the health services, and then only superficially.

Every theory of organization formed since the Second World War, for instance, has something to say about the need for people to feel valued at work. Frederick Herzberg's motivation theory goes as far as to state that after a certain level, money is a less important consideration for people than receiving recognition and appreciation for their work and having opportunities for growth and development (Pugh & Hickson 1989). Yet every year, when the pay review bodies are ready to deliver their reports, there is a national outcry about who gets paid how much, by whom, and for doing what. Money has become a surrogate for all those things that we just cannot seem to get from the job – unconditional respect, progression, fringe benefits, recognition, and time to dream.

In health care there have always been difficult decisions to make about pay, services, costs and staffing levels. In days gone by, few staff would have been directly involved in them; someone else, somewhere else, was always there to carry the burden. Now, every healthcare worker is touched by the uncertainties that other organizations face – limited financial resources, fragmenting societies, increasing demand for services, a shrinking pool of relevant skills, more educated and knowledgeable users, an explosion in information technology applications, and an ever-more chaotic world.

On the face of it, this should mean that leaders have never had it so good. Uncertainty and chaos are exactly the circumstances that have, in the past, produced superb leaders – people who can create order out of chaos, who can bring enough clarity to the mess to convince people that there is a 'right way' to proceed. But looking at it another way, leaders have never had it so bad. Uncertainty creates imbalance in every part of our lives. Alvin Tofler's *Future Shock* (Tofler 1985) gave advance warning about what happens when people face several changes at once – they want to opt for the seemingly simple solutions. Leaders who do not provide these simple solutions are criticized, despised, or worse.

It is therefore not surprising that, for all the theory, the practice of leadership is often the exercise of the quick-fix solution, aimed at pleasing the largest number for the shortest time. Doing something – *anything* – makes us feel better, and less at the mercy of Fate. Our leaders, at our behest, oblige by assuring us that the crisis is over, security restored, and the sun will always shine. We collude, and our serial problems pile up. Eventually, another crisis occurs, and the cycle repeats.

The NHS has tended to manage the numerous changes in its organization and operation in this 'sticking-plaster' approach to problem-solving and decision-making. And it works – but only up to a point.

SUPPORT YOUR LOCAL LEADER

Being a leader can be lonely. When I worked as a director of a department in an NHS Regional Health Authority (RHA), I would stay in my office long after everyone else had gone home. I used the time to catch up on reading, answer e-mail, or just wind down. I also took stock of what I had accomplished that day, gaining a rather one-sided view in the process, but who else was there to ask?

Managers and leaders rarely get praised to their face, except under exceptional circumstances. Yet a well-timed 'thank you' or 'well done' can go a long way to boosting the confidence of the most ego-laden person. To be effective, leaders need supportive environments. Theoretically, this includes the right to make mistakes, peer learning, time to think and learn, supportive colleagues, and time to play.

At the first ever forum of healthcare chief executives in 1997, these well-paid, seemingly powerful and aware individuals confessed to feeling 'powerless to influence the national health policy agenda' (Butler 1997). I confess to having feelings of cynicism on first reading that story. After all, if this (predominantly male) group of healthcare leaders, with the power to terminate employment, services and self-esteem, felt powerless, what must healthcare assistants be feeling, and where is their forum? But on the tenth reading, something struck home. *They were waiting for a lead*. These chief executives had discovered that there is a limit to positional power.

Many organizational theories emphasize this point – positional power is self-limiting (Pfeffer 1992). Personal power (or influence), on the other hand, is not. But if most of your day is spent meeting crises, where do you find the time to build personal power? Power unused evaporates (Larsen 1988). Can we learn how to 'grow' leaders, and can we develop new ways of being leaders which do not stop us from being productive?

From her research on what current healthcare chief executives say they need to grow and develop, Fritchie has identified four key needs – moving beyond, extending and expanding, keeping afloat, and deepening and developing (Fritchie 1997).

1. *Moving beyond* concerns change, testing choices, testing alternatives, and reflecting. The possibilities to achieve these aims include job swaps, shadowing, secondment, and biography workshops.
2. In *extending and expanding*, leaders seek different ways to use all their skills, not just those immediately required by the job. Possibilities here include consultancy, non-executive roles, mentoring, project work.
3. Leaders who want to *deepen and develop* their skills may be fulfiled by educational programmes (MBA, leadership development, specialist seminars). This type of development requires intensive planning, resources and support, both internally and externally.
4. *Keeping afloat* is the most basic level of development. Issues such as time management and media training would be part of this development process. Personal pursuits (walking, gardening, hobbies in general) are also vital in helping leaders keep their heads above water.

Regardless of the organizational position that leaders hold, they all need this range of development opportunities. Research suggests that the more junior the organizational position of the leaders, the more they will need support and development. It is puzzling, therefore, to find that organizations spend a disproportionate amount of money on the development process of the few senior staff that they have.

Fritchie's research in the NHS suggested such a bias in the NHS. The focus of her work was growing leaders and trying to identify the kind of opportunities they required to develop, but the results showed that most of the attention was given to chief executives, or those aspiring to such roles. What will happen if we don't apply effort to finding leader 'saplings', and only work hard on already established plants? It is unlikely that we will produce the contrasts that make so many gardens attractive and interesting if we continue to pursue these policies.

It is nonsense to focus so much on the apex of any organization. To be realistic, an organization can survive up to 2 years without a chief executive. Some organizations are even considering abolishing the post altogether and moving to more collegiate, collaborative models of working. Certainly, many fast-developing entrepreneurial companies do not have chief executives, or even managers as we know them. But *every* company needs leaders.*

THE DOWNSIDE – I WANT TO GO HOME

Learning about the downside of leading shouldn't necessarily depress you. On the contrary, if you have a clear sense of your potentials and limitations and can therefore be realistic about your goals, you are more likely to become a successful and effective leader.

You'll be familiar with the expression, 'biting off more than you can chew'? Just like the elephant-eaters described in Chapter 1, leaders must only take on as much as they can realistically achieve. There is no shame in this. It is not 'giving up' or 'throwing in the towel', it is not running away from the problem – it is being honest with self and others. You might be thinking that people have every right to hold legitimate expectations of what leaders will do with and for them, and I wouldn't argue with you. But leaders also have rights, one of which is the right not to wander down the path to oblivion by committing themselves to meet *other people's* expectations. And they also have the responsibility not to mislead people who chose to or want to follow them.

Think about the leaders you have learnt the most from. Their accomplishments may seem truly stupendous – almost superhuman. They might seem responsible for achieving the most marvellous things. But think again. Is it possible that much of their success was down to an ability to get the maximum output from the minimum input? In other words, were they not brilliant practitioners of the essential skill called 'leverage'?

How finely honed are your leverage skills? Even if you are single, have no family or friends immediately around you, eat little, sleep little, and have enough money to have others shop, clean and cook for you, the day is only as long as you are able to function effectively in it. Forget about being superhuman. Focus on being *fully* human. Resist your humanity and you

---

*In the 1980s, many entrepreneurial companies especially in the computer industry, were in disarray because they had no management structures. We all sit back and applaud when we hear of some entrepreneurial knight in shining armour who so bravely slays the dragons of bureaucracy, inefficiency, and humbug. Frankly, bureaucracies serve a purpose – someone has to pay the bills, maintain the premises, and generally ensure that the business keeps within the relevant laws. When it doesn't happen, chaos – and bankruptcy – reign. Entrepreneurs do not make good managers. They are much better at enthusing people than at managing them. As for leadership – well, they don't always succeed here either. Too often they succumb to hubris, arrogance, and a belief in their seeming omnipotence. Don't believe everything you read in the papers about these heroic figures. Remember that leadership, like reflection, often occurs out of the limelight, and with little fanfare.

are likely to be forever disappointed with yourself and with others. Give in to your humanness, and fashion your leadership from that base.

HUMANNESS AND EMOTION – FIT FOR PURPOSE?

Yet humanness is not a quality universally admired in the health services. For some, it is too closely aligned to that dreaded word 'emotion'. Surely, they argue, there is no place for emotion in leadership? Surely the intrusion of emotion would make the activity of leadership, which requires a dispassionate and objective perspective, almost impossible to carry out? I beg to differ.

One of the great mysteries of contemporary health care is why we ever allowed ourselves to believe that we must keep emotion out of our work. To deny the inherent emotion in health care is to deny our common humanity with our patients. Someone once said that to understand others we need to understand how they operate as meaning-creating creatures, how we each experience ourselves and our world. To put it more simply, if not as elegantly, we need to walk a mile in another's shoes before we can begin to understand their view of the world. If we also deny our common humanity with colleagues, with whom we generally share a common language, then we cannot ever have productive, enhancing relationships with people who are other than us, and depend on us for care, protection, and healing. In denying emotion, we deny reality.

I had to learn about this the hard way. In the late 1970s I was healthy, bursting with energy, slept little, loved my job, and looked forward to the future. Then I became ill. A 'routine' operation for appendicitis caused complications, and I was hospitalized for 3 weeks. One night, tucked up in my single room away from the main ward, I awoke to hear someone crying in the single room next to mine. It was a woman, and she seemed to cry for a long time. I wanted to go to her but could not. I rang for the night staff who took, to me, a long time to arrive. I told the staff nurse that the woman next door seemed upset about something. I shall never forget her remark: 'Oh, she had an abortion. Anyway, if she wants anything she knows to ring the bell'. She then walked away.

That was one of the few times in my life that I wanted to do real violence to someone. The nurse seemed to have given up on the woman at a time when she most needed care. I don't want to get into the issue of caring, except to say that leaders understand the difference between professional attention to a need (in the nurse's case, administering medical care), and caring (the giving of compassion). Leaders care, long after their professional attention is required.

WATCHING AND LEARNING

While in hospital, I began to question such practices as routinely giving staff who were admitted as patients, side rooms away from the main ward. I developed a suspicion that this had less to do with showing courtesy (and not a little favouritism) to a fellow-professional, and more about ensuring that prying and potentially critical eyes were not cast over the practices on the unit. More recent experience of inpatient services has only deepened this suspicion. Realizations such as these did not change my behaviour overnight, but gradually I became more questioning and even more reluctant to do as I was told and 'know my place'.

My life certainly changed, but it was so gradual that it was a long time before I was conscious of how much. The most obvious difference was the way in which I treated patients, and how I viewed nursing. Patients gradually became less of an intrusion into my daily practice, as I used to see it. Nursing was re-established for me as an art, aided and abetted by science. The emotional side of caring became more important which, it has to be said, made my job much more stressful. It was during this time of professional re-birth that I began to be interested in the operations of the wider organization I worked in.

Before this, I had hardly noticed the managers who ran the hospital. They were just there, making little or no impact on my life, or so I thought. If I felt strongly enough about something I would speak out, but for most of the time I, like most of my colleagues, got on with the job. Does this sound familiar? It took the drama of a hospital fire to shake me out of my apathy, and enable me for the first time to consciously notice how some managers behave.

This was probably the most frightening experience of my life, and even writing about it now makes me feel uncomfortable. A confused elderly woman in one of the four bed bays of the ward set fire to her bed in the early morning. One of my colleagues was taking a break, and the other was attending to an elderly man in another part of the ward. Smelling smoke, I hurried down the corridor and saw what I thought was a dim light on in one of the bays. Of the two women in the room, the one nearer the door had her leg in traction. The other, next to a door which opened onto a garden, was barely visible through thickening smoke.

I cannot tell you exactly what I did, but in a short time, the woman with traction was in the corridor, still in bed, and I was physically lifting the other from her bed, wrapped in a sheet, and was pulling her along the floor into the corridor. The next definite memory I have is of standing in the garden with a smouldering mattress at my feet, and shivering. I was also aware that someone wearing red was talking to me in quite a harsh voice. Next, a familiar face was next to me, and someone was hugging me and gently leading me away from the ward.

It was some hours before I had the full story. The light I had seen was the lit match which had set the bed alight. Apparently, after going into the room I had set off the fire alarm, pulled the first bed into the corridor, pulled the woman from her smoking bed and dragged her into the corridor, and then gone back into the room and shoved the smoking mattress out of the door.

Those particular mattresses emitted cyanide gas when they burned. When the fire brigade arrived, the officer in charge had yelled at me (that was the harsh voice) for tackling the mattress after moving the patients. I want to believe that his reaction was due to fear, because fires in hospitals are no fun for the fire service. The person who did the hugging was the matron who had been called from home and had arrived, serene and unflappable, perfectly dressed and made-up. You notice such things when you are stressed. She was concerned about my reaction to the fire officer, with whom she found me in a fury when she arrived. The hug certainly stopped the shivering. I also felt that it validated my action, even though I had not acted in complete compliance with the fire policy then in operation.

There was also a third manager who impressed himself on me – the doctor who looked after the elderly woman in whose bed the fire started. She was transferred to another hospital, where she subsequently died from pneumonia and heart failure. This doctor spent much time over a period of weeks reassuring me that nothing I had done was in any way responsible for her death. It was several months before I gave myself permission to believe him. But I also had to reassure others – the woman's relatives were devastated because they had given her the matches which caused the fire. They felt guilty, and wanted forgiveness from the staff.

Shortly after that incident, I became much more interested in management issues, and how people behaved toward each other at work. The three manager figures had acted differently, depending on their perception of their role in the incident and their belief in my competence. The matron became an early role model, especially in terms of compassion. I learnt a valuable lesson from the fire officer – rules exist for a purpose – and from the doctor about not giving up on people – you cannot change how someone feels about themselves, but you can help by remaining positive about the possibility that they *can* change.

This talk of leaders and how they can exhibit different behaviours and different personalities leads me inevitably to *Star Trek*.

STAR TREK CAPTAINS DO IT IN DEEP SPACE

Without overdoing it, I believe that *Star Trek* can teach us many things about leadership, not least of which is the fact that different circumstances create different kinds of leaders. I want to discuss *Star Trek* in some detail because the models of leaders and leadership it presents are of relevance to health care.

Clearly, the phenomenon that is *Star Trek* serves a purpose for many people, and not just because of the uniforms. *Star Trek*'s emergence coincides with the time when the cry went up for leaders of vision and integrity, and it has continued to move (or should we say, 'boldly go'?) with the times. It is as if *Star Trek*, the experiment in a new type of science fiction programming that was initially not as successful as imagined, has become a laboratory where, under the safe conditions of a studio set, ideas can run riot.

The macho Captain Kirk, original leader and inspiration of the starship *Enterprise*, was succeeded by the urbane, diplomatic, almost phlegmatic Picard, who was European to boot. It is quite appropriate that Picard's crew are called the *Next Generation*, different from the original in every way. A new world of Starfleet settings was created with *Deep Space Nine (DS9)*, and the post-modern *Voyager*.

It is interesting that Jean Luc Picard remains the most loved *Star Trek* captain. Aloof, unemotional, wise, trenchant, caring and complex, he presents a do-not-mess-with-me persona which gives his crew a feeling of safety. No Kirk-like encounters with evil damsels in weird clothes, and even weirder hair. Captain Picard is the omnipotent figure many of us look for in a leader. He even has a school of leadership named after his call sign – 'Make it So'. However, he would probably not survive on *DS9*, the station which goes nowhere.

DS9's captain, Sisko, spent the first series in emotional pain over the loss of his wife. Constable Odo silently leaks emotion like a sieve because he knows no other of his kind. The Bajoran first office, Kira, shoots sparks every time she opens her mouth, Doctor Bashir is tense, Chief Engineer O'Brien expects every ship to be like the *Enterprise* (where he managed the transporter system), and the Ferengi who runs the bar on the station is a rogue who despises 'hu-mans'. Sisko's chief of operation is Worf the Klingon, he of the humourless stare. Dax the Trill, the cerebral and sensual science officer, completes this crew. Emotion is everywhere on *DS9* – from Sisko and his need for a female presence in his and his son's life, to Dax and Worf who are 'an item'.

The skill of the writers and producers of *Star Trek* is such that the science is real and plausible, and so are the situations and how they are dealt with. Let me give you an example. While writing this chapter, I took a break and watched a taped episode of *DS9*. The storyline was about a Klingon general, blind in one eye, who is asked to lead a mission to rescue a Klingon starship. Worf goes along as his first officer, and Dax as science officer.

Now, the bridge of a Klingon warship is not like your average starship. Discipline is rigid. At the beginning of each mission, the crew pledge their lives to the captain, who in turn, is asked to keep them safe and lead them to victory. On this particular ship, the crew are demoralized after losing several battles to the Jem'Hadar, a group of warriors who are programmed to fight. To cut a long story short, Worf decides to relieve the captain of his command for failing to lead the crew into battle. The captain is shaken from his apathy by this apparent mutiny and in the subsequent fight, wins the battle with the Jem'Hadar, rescues the trapped Klingons, and then they all get commendations from the Klingon High Council.

Like most episodes of *Star Trek*, there is a moral. This time it concerned the dilemma of doing what is ordered, or doing what is *right*. Back in the real world, there are echoes of this dilemma in David Seedhouse's theory of 'everyday ethics', in which he argues that rather that trying to twist our brains round abstract definitions of concepts such as 'ethics' and 'morals', it is the almost intuitive, common or 'everyday' ethics we hold dear which offer the most appropriate guide to help us deal with real-life dilemmas and tensions (Seedhouse 1988). In this case, the dilemma is whether we should do things simply because they are ordered. Everyday ethics requires us to question how appropriate, how *right*, the order is for the circumstances.

The concept of everyday ethics is also central to the plight of the crew of the starship *Voyager*. First of all, the captain is a woman, Kathryn Janeway. Sure enough, she has received a rough press. She is too soft, does not take decisions. She allows her crew to argue with her. And so on.

Voyager's circumstances are very different from the other vessels in the series – an unhappy encounter with an Entity (a highly technologically advanced alien known as the Caretaker) blasts them into the Delta quadrant for outside Federation air space, from which it will take them 70 years to get home. The crew of the *Voyager* is composed of bona fide Starfleet officers, and misfits – most of whom are Starfleet training school drop-outs, not considered fit to wear the uniform.

The *Voyager* crew is saturated with emotion, and face a range of ethical conflicts which are different in both quality and range from that faced by their colleagues. For example, how to manage one consequence of personal relationships between crew members – babies. On the one hand, the babies will grow up and some (or all) will join the crew. On the other hand, is it right to raise children in the artificial environment of a starship? The crews on the *Enterprise* and *DS9* go back to earth often. The *Voyager* crew does not have that option. But Captain Janeway has other ethical dilemmas.

The Prime Directive (*Star Trek* code of conduct) is not recognized inside the Delta quadrant. But Janeway refuses to let a little thing like being adrift in an unknown and potentially hostile quadrant stop her from adhering to the tenets of the Prime Directive. In fact, it was adherence to the moral and ethical principles of the Prime Directive that got them lost in the first place – the Entity (the Caretaker) could have been defeated, but that would have meant the destruction of a vulnerable population who had been dependent on the Entity. That some of her senior staff oppose Janeway's position, does not easily sway her. For Janeway, the fact that they are in unfamiliar territory is precisely why the Prime Directive must not be nullified – it is the code that provides a moral guide for the crew, one they all understand.

To reject Janeway's leadership style because she is not Picard/Sisko/

Kirk is to ignore a fundamental issue about leaders – they emerge to suit the circumstances in which they find themselves. The bottom line is how effective are they in doing the primary job of a leader, which is to get consistent performance from people – voluntarily. By that criterion, all the leaders in *Star Trek* are *leaders*. Their *personalities* are different, but they portray the adaptive ability of all effective leaders, and are all excellent at scanning the future.

You can draw similar conclusions from how leaders in different positions in organizations respond to their environment. At the clinical level, the present is the overriding factor – do I have enough resources, what is the workload likely to be, will everyone show up for work? As you take on more general management tasks, the future takes greater precedence – will we be giving the same range of services in the next 2 years, what range of skills will we need to stay effective and successful, how do we develop our future leaders? Kouzes and Posner suggest that the factor which differentiates 'tactical' leaders from 'strategic' leaders is the amount of time spent on looking into the future (Kouzes and Posner 1995). Tactical leaders are more oriented to the present, while strategic leaders are oriented to the future.

Well, that is how it should be, and we need both kinds of leaders. But the reality is that less than 3% of senior managers spend any time on future-gazing. Does that mean that 97+% of senior managers are working tactically? If so, with what effect? If most managers are doing tactics, who is dreaming about, and longing to create, the future? Do you?

TIME OUT

A 1994 article in *Fortune* magazine relates the stories of several leaders who stepped off the corporate treadmill, with the blessing of their organizations (Sherman 1994). Many US business schools are now including 'reflection' as part of required course work, and major companies are teaching their staff how to be introspective. If you are tempted to scoff at these initiatives, consider for a moment how many times at work you have wished that you had just a little time to think about what you were doing, to consider alternatives? Reflection is part of continuous learning – act, reflect, learn, move on.

But time to think requires an environment which validates taking time to think. Remember the story in Chapter 1, about the care of the elderly ward that was closed over a Christmas period, but the decision was not communicated to key people? That was a result of people *not* taking time to think, even in the short term.

A constant complaint from nurses is that there is little time to reflect on how we practise. The health service is run on an 'action' model which often leads to exhaustion, poor decision-making and poor communication. Well, I am offering you time to think now. Take time out now and write down three things that you want to see change in how you practise nursing. You may want to use the following questions as an aid in this exercise:

- How much time can I commit to making the change I want to see?
- Am I the right person to implement this change?
- What impact will this change have on others?
- Why do I want this change?

Sometimes we have to practise taking time out, so that time out can become part of our practice.

READING ABOUT LEADERSHIP VERSUS DOING IT

Reading about a topic in which you are interested is one way to learn about it. But what should you read about leadership? If you want to read about leadership, first decide what it is you want to know, confirm, or are just curious about. As a simple rule of thumb, books on leadership should have the following properties; they should:

- be written in simple language
- have applications to the real world
- be easily available
- not use 'he/him' as a catch-all term for both sexes
- have jokes, cartoons, stories, and other non-academic stuff
- not be too heavy to carry.

These are survival tips, because there are as many books on leadership as there are leaders living, and to be born. Many appear to be ego trips. Others are just off the wall. Still others can instil an inferiority complex faster than a Formula 1 driver can do a lap.

People who write books about leadership come in many forms. Avoid those which glow in the dark – usually a sign that they have been lit from within by hubris. In all honesty, all you need to know about leadership, you know already. The books should be used as reference sources to guide and challenge you. Some of the best books are fun to read, and are moderately irreverent, not to mention having really good jokes. Authors like Charles Handy use plain English, dry humour, and pull no punches. Other titles such as *Leadership Secrets of Attila the Hun*, and *Victory Secrets of Attila the Hun* not only entertain, but put ideas across in a thoughtful way, and are full of the kind of maxims which can be useful at those times when you cannot quite find the right words, e.g. 'The essence of risk-taking is acting without the assurance that you have all the relevant facts'.

This is not to say that more academic texts are not valuable. Authors such as Rosabeth Moss Kanter present research on leadership in a straightforward way that encourages you to turn the page. And this is probably the key. Like any good book, the story must excite, stir, and ultimately make you care about what happens to the characters. All good books on leadership have that element. I cannot tell you what to read. However, whatever you do read remember – we can become what we read.

Inappropriate reading nearly led to my own demise as a leader. I was a strong believer in the concept of the leader who builds morale, corrals the troops, and heads off in the direction they believe to be right. I did not give enough consideration to the fact that people have to want to be followers. I had a job to do, and I set out to conquer. Instead, I almost destroyed my self-confidence because I missed a key signal – one of my followers was my manager, and she had a different set of priorities.

I failed to listen, I failed to ask questions, I failed to hear warnings, and I failed to find a fall-back position. The result was a period of low self-esteem, self-doubt about my ability to lead, and lack of self-confidence in my competence as a practitioner. The books do not prepare you for this, and they cannot.

After my near calamity, I started taking more notice of the live leaders I worked with, one of whom was my manager (yes, the one who triggered my distress). I noticed how open and direct she was with the staff, how she attached herself to their concerns, without losing her authority. I also noticed how much respect she engendered, without necessarily being liked – she *was* liked, she just did not have a *need* to be liked.

The most valuable lesson I learnt from this period of my life was how to recover from failure. In Chapter 8 we will look in detail at the reasons why leaders fail. For now, consider this: leaders fail when they stop thinking, and when they stop taking the actions they need to succeed.

NURSES AS LEADERS

Nurses can, and do, succeed as leaders. For a long time, however, we have been more managed than led, and such leadership as there has been has tended to be poor. Interestingly, nurses who are successful leaders do not recognize themselves as such. Remember Alison Mennie's story in Chapter 2? She called herself a pleb! This is not unusual language from a member of an occupational group whose status is low compared with others. But if we change the way we speak about our success, that may be a good starting place from which to increase the visibility of our leaders.

The Royal College of Nursing's (RCN) Ward Leadership has started this process (Cunningham 1997). The focus of the RCN's programme is improving patient care. From the comments of participants, what they value most about the programme is the way it legitimizes the time they spend talking to patients. Leaders such as these can therefore begin to lead us all back to the reason why the NHS exists – because people need care.

Nurses work at all levels and in all areas of health care. Our ubiquity should give us maximum leverage in terms of leadership. But how do we exercise this leverage? Let us start by cleaning up our language.

LEADING AND LANGUAGE

In every staff attitude survey I have ever seen, 'poor communication' is always in the top five factors that employees believe make the workplace less enjoyable than say, repeat episodes of Brookside. (Curiously, 'money' rarely features in the top 20). Unfortunately, these surveys tend not to explore the specifics, such as how often staff get praised for their work, or how they find out about changes in the organization. Nor do they ask questions that relate to the type of language used in the organization.

All words convey meaning, meanings which are often dependent on what you want to say, to whom you want to say it, and what you want to achieve by saying it. When we speak, therefore, we have to be clear not only about what we are saying, but also about the words we have chosen to convey the meaning.

Let me give an example. You want to introduce a change in the way patients are booked for admission to your ward. You want to decrease their level of distress on admission, and give your colleagues more time to talk with patients and plan their care. The language you choose to express this desire for change is likely to be positive, articulating the benefits to patients and nurses. But as a leader you have followers, and some are not convinced. One colleague begins to exhibit signs of a type of behaviour which all too frequently raises its ugly head when change feels threatening – a behaviour I call 'The Drain'. It consists mainly of saying why such and such will not work, and why nothing can be done about it anyway. It drenches your positive idea in gloom, and pours your inspiration down the drain of despair. If there is enough 'drain behaviour', your plans may have to be shelved, or revised. That is not a problem because your vision has to be shared and tested, allowing others to amend and refine it. But people acting like Drains do not want to share – they want to give up.

The phrases they use are an indication of this desire:

- It won't work.
- We can't change anything.
- They won't let us do that.
- If only we had (followed by a wistful wish list), we could do it.
- I'm too old for all this.

And so on. The above phrases are *reactive*, that is, they are negative responses to circumstances. Contrast that to the colleagues who, while also sceptical, are willing to take on the challenge:

- Let us think about another way to do this.

- Who has done something similar? Who can we copy?
- How can we sell the idea so we get what we need?
- It could work if we …
- Let us ask the patients what they think.

When facing a challenge, which set of phrases are you more likely to use? The challenge can be in your personal, work, or social life. If you have a tendency to be *reactive* to circumstances, reflect on why that might be. Do not give yourself a hard time if that is the case. However, if you want to fully develop your potential as a leader, you need to consider how the words you chose to talk about what you want to do can make or break your vision. Listen carefully to the people who energize and inspire you. The words and phrases they use are more than likely to be *proactive* rather than reactive.

Look at the set of phrases in Exercise 4.1. Against each put the letter *R* if you thing it is reactive, and the letter *P* if you think the phrase is proactive.

Exercise 4.1

- I prefer
- I don't want to
- I can't
- I can do that
- I choose
- I can control my feelings
- She makes me so mad
- I have to do that
- They told me to
- There is no alternative
- I don't know how you do that

- We need to make a decision
- I must …
- Can we try another way?
- I can create an alternative
- Make it so
- They won't let me
- I shall
- It's all the same to me
- Follow me
- We won!

If we want to win as leaders, we have to start by choosing winning words – words that define us as a powerful occupational group, with a key and definable role to play in the planning, delivery, monitoring and development of health care. One of the most telling marks of others' perceptions of us as a large but relatively powerless group is our continued inability to protect the resources we need to treat our patients safely, effectively and efficiently. We always seem to finally find our voice and speak out, but too often, it is after the damage has been done.

We can do no better than look to the example of Florence Nightingale as someone who was able to use language effectively to get things done.

Contrary to the 'Lady with the Lamp' image, Florence Nightingale was no shrinking violet. For over 4 decades she manoeuvred, manipulated, orchestrated and generally made merry hell for those she saw as not following her lead.

Like her contemporary, Mary Seacole (see Chapter 2), Nightingale rarely took 'no' as the final word on anything. She saw an urgent need to improve radically the medical care of soldiers in the Crimea and promptly set about making her views known. It did not matter that few wanted to hear. She kept on talking – proactively, powerfully – and acted.

If Nightingale were living today we might find her less than agreeable. But though her message and teachings speak to nurses of all times, she was very much a woman of her own times. Like all great leaders, she emerged to recognize, challenge and match the circumstances of her age.

Nurses today have greater opportunities than ever before to lead health care. Some, however, may view these opportunities as threats to their internalized view of themselves as powerless, lacking influence, excluded from important decisions. But unless we speak up and speak out, no one will know we have a view, much less a stake in the future of health care. You do not have to be a firebrand, charismatic, heroic type of leader. Other quieter characteristics are probably more important, as we will discuss in the next chapter.

Key learning points

- To succeed, leaders need support – from peers, as well as from the organization.

- How words/phrases are used can make or break leaders.

- 'Emotion' is not a dirty word.

- Reading about leadership can seriously damage your well being. Choose carefully.

- Taking time to think is not time wasted.

- Nurses are leaders too.

- Using reactive or proactive words is a matter of choice.

REFERENCES

Butler P 1997 It's tough at the top. Health Service Journal, 6 November: 12–13
Cunningham G 1997 Ward leadership. Nursing Standard, 12(4): 20–25
Fritchie R 1997 How to grow leaders. Health Service Journal, 6 November: 12–13
Kouzes J, Posner B 1995 The leadership challenge: how to keep getting extraordinary things done in organizations. Jossey-Bass, San Francisco

Larsen J 1988 Being powerful: talk into action. In: White R (ed) Political issues in nursing: past, present and future, vol 3. John Wiley, Chichester

Pfeffer J 1992 Managing with power. Harvard Business School Press, Boston

Pugh D S, Hickson D J 1989 Writers on organizations, 4th edn. Penguin, London

Seedhouse D 1988 Ethics: the heart of health care. John Wiley, Chichester

Sherman S 1994 Leaders learn to heed the voice within. Fortune, 130:4

Tofler A 1985 Future Shock. Pan, London

5

So you want to be a leader?

Key words:

characteristics of leaders; self-evaluation; environmental audit

In this chapter, I want to focus on some of the basics of leadership. Exactly how can you tell effective leaders from the rest? Can we learn to be effective leaders? If so, what skills do we need? Until we find the gene for leadership (I hope that is a joke), we will have to use the tools we already have – our experience of effective leaders, our values and beliefs, and our instinct.

You probably already have an identikit image of your ideal leader. You probably try to emulate this person, be as like them as possible. Leaders are ordinary people who achieve extraordinary things. It is the personal characteristics that lead them to achieve the extraordinary that we will look at in the first half of this chapter.

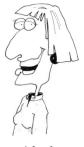

A leader

In the second half, you will have the opportunity to complete self-evaluation activities based on four key characteristics of leadership: power, life position, networking, and homework. You will also have the chance to assess your current working environment in terms of how it supports your development as a leader. Remember not to berate yourself if you find deficiencies in your progress; focus instead on what you need to learn and practise to become a more effective leader. At the end of all the exercises I will give you some more tips on how to get the support you need.

MADE TO MEASURE

Try Exercise 5.1:

Exercise 5.1

1. Write down 10 essential characteristics you would want to find in a leader.

2. Allocate 10 points to each characteristic.

3. Against each characteristic, write the names of five people you know who consistently exhibit this attribute.

4. Share the 10 points allocated to each characteristic between each person.

5. Total their scores and place them in rank order.

6. When you have finished, reflect on the following questions:

   ● Why did you choose those particular characteristics?

   ● Are your chosen leaders mainly male, mainly female, or a mixture of both?

   ● Were your choices of leaders from nursing, or from other backgrounds (family, friends, etc.)?

   ● Did you put yourself on the list?

I did the exercise, and felt uncomfortable when I wrote my name against my chosen characteristics. But by not recognizing the leadership potential within ourselves, we are half-way towards setting ourselves up to fail as leaders. It is a curious but true fact that many of the people we believe to be leaders do not consider themselves as such, so we are not alone in this lack of self-awareness. Later, we will look in more detail at some of the other things leaders do not always consciously know about themselves. For now, let us focus on those obvious characteristics which mark effective leaders.

CHARACTERISTICS OF EFFECTIVE LEADERS

I have selected 13 characteristics, based on observation and experience, and placed them in three categories: communication and language, behaviour, and development. The full list is set out in Box 5.1. Notice that the majority of characteristics concern the behaviours through which certain values are expressed.

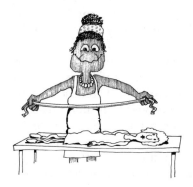

Made to measure

Box 5.1   Characteristics of effective leaders

Communication and language
1. Proactive language
2. Use jargon only when necessary
3. Listen

Behaviour
4. The 5 'F' words: friendly, fun, focused, flexible, fast
5. Trust
6. Values
7. Passion
8. Integrity and honesty
9. Politically savvy
10. Productive life position
11. Use of power

Development
12. Homework
13. Networking

You may expand the list of characteristics if you want to, but remember that they must be related to *performance*. 'Not hurting people's feelings' is a reasonable characteristic, but it might not contribute to a leader's effectiveness.

Communication and language

Effective leaders are proactive. Being proactive means more than taking the initiative. It also encompasses the notion of 'response-ability', or acting responsibly and positively. Being annoyed about things we do not like is understandable, but a leader has to be able to direct the energy generated by the emotion of annoyance into positive action. Simply sitting, seething, and tiring yourself out by rehearsing over and over again what you would like to say or do, isn't really an option for the proactive leader.

Language is linked to proactivity because words are maps to our inner world; they indicate how we perceive what happens, and how we formulate a response. Look again at the list of reactive and proactive phrases in Chapter 4 (Exercise 4.1, p. 62). Proactive words and phrases reveal choice and response-ability. Reactive words reflect the perception of not being in control. But you can still choose to respond reactively to circumstances, if you feel that is the appropriate response in the circumstances. Stephen Covey's Circle of Concern and Circle of Influence illustrate how proactive and reactive responses can influence action (see Fig. 5.1) (Covey 1999).

In the Circle of Concern are those things over which we have little control. The Circle of Influence consists of those things we can do something about. The amount of energy and time we spend on each circle depends on whether we perceive ourselves as response-able, or at the mercy of others. Effective leaders work to increase their Circle of Influence, inside and outside the workplace, which means that effective leaders are also effective people. Later in this chapter, there will be an opportunity for you to consider which of the circles you expend most of your energy on.

Effective leaders use jargon only when necessary. The *Oxford Concise Dictionary* has two main listings for jargon. One is: 'words or expressions used by a particular group or profession; gibberish; debased or barbarous language'. The other reads: 'a translucent, colourless, or smoky variety of zircon' (I love dictionaries). Think of the leaders you have known. Which of these definitions would best describe how they talk about what they are doing, and what they want you to do?

One thing in which the health service excels is inappropriate use of jargon. Whether it is used as a sword to eliminate 'undesirables' from the decision-making process, or as a shield to hide managers' fears, insecurities, ignorance, failure, and feelings of inadequacy, you don't have to look far to find jargon.

Effective leaders do not mask their goals by wrapping them up in unnecessary jargon. They are more likely to use painfully clear and plain language, which is the essence of good communication. You will not find

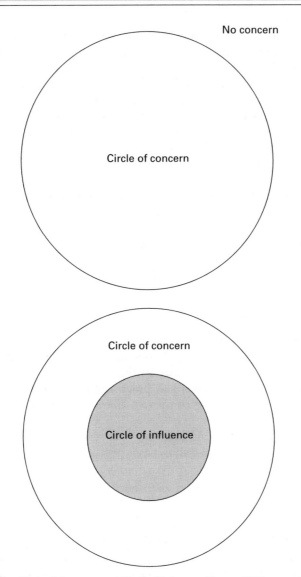

Figure 5.1   The Circle of Concern and Circle of Influence (Covey 1999, reproduced by permission of the publisher, Simon & Schuster Ltd, © Stephen R. Covey 1989).

effective leaders talking about the need to 'rightsize the organization', or 'create a strategic intent to maximize our potential in the marketplace of the future'. The first means sacking people, the second is gibberish. And you can hear such 'dirty talk' everyday in some organizations where people are struggling to understand their part in achieving 'our overarching vision for transforming our capacity to meet the global challenges of the marketplace for the 21st century and beyond'. Effective leaders neither tolerate nor use language like this. Calling a spade a digging implement is not part of an effective leader's vocabulary.

Effective leaders listen. You will have to search long and hard to find an effective leader who does not know how to listen. Like all healthcare professionals, nurses are taught about communicating with patients early in their careers. So why is it that, year after year, the Parliamentary Commissioner for Administration's (the Ombudsman) annual report about investigations into patients' complaints cites 'communication with staff as the major cause of dissatisfaction with care? The classic complaint that 'everybody tells me something different' is still commonly cited.

I once had responsibility for monitoring Patient's Charter standards across a London RHA, and the Ombudsman's reports about complaints formed part of my attempts to improve the way in which patients received and obtained information. As a still practising midwife, I also see at first hand how not listening causes confusion, distress, worry, and can endanger lives.

Listening is more than just hearing. It is responding appropriately to what is heard. Look at the two short cases presented in Box 5.2.

Box 5.2 Cases

Case 1
Miss J. is admitted to hospital for assessment as she has had several falls at home. When she gets to the ward, she is interviewed by two nurses, one a tutor. Roper's model of care is used to create a care plan for Miss J. The interview lasts for about 90 minutes. For most of that time, Miss J. seems distracted, which the nurses surmise is part of her confusion about being in hospital. At the end of the interview, Miss J. is asked if she had any particular concerns about being in hospital. In reply she says 'Who is going to look after my cat'? That worry was the cause of her distraction, but the question was never asked until the end of the interview.

Case 2
Mr R. needs to have a series of tests to investigate his recent falls. He says he understands exactly what will happen to him, but he asks the same question over and over again: 'How much time will I have to take off work?' He never receives a satisfactory answer – the staff concentrate so much on his medical problems, they fail to recognize the issue which is worrying Mr R. *most* – possibly losing his job through prolonged absence.

In both cases, it is obvious these two people are very anxious about being in hospital. Too often we *hear* such anxiety, but do not really *listen* to it. We arrive at our conclusion about what people's main concerns *should* be, and don't listen to what they *actually* are. We have our own anxieties constantly in mind to muddy the waters even further – about resources, our own frailty, being tired, or having to deal with personal problems. There are times when it seems to me that for some of us, patients get in the way of the work. If only they were not so needy. I believe that nurses will not realize their full potential as leaders unless we learn to listen with our hearts as well as our ears.

Behaviour

Effective leaders use the 'F' words. This isn't as vulgar as it sounds! Rosabeth Moss Kanter defined the 'F' words that are so important to good leadership – friendly, fun, focused, flexible, and fast (Alimo-Metcalfe 1993). They have *fast* reactions to change, encourage innovation, and have a questioning mentality. Leaders are *focused* on specific goals, which are owned by everyone. They create a *friendly* environment which supports collaboration, enthusiasm and commitment from staff and other 'stakeholders'. Leaders are *flexible*, using their own and everyone else's skills to the limit. Not least, they create a *fun* place to work.

Of all the 'F' words, fun and friendliness must be joint-top of the list. In these times of scarce resources, short-term contracts and 60-hour working weeks, who wants a leader who is a humourless killjoy? Oh, all right. They are all over your organization like a rash. So why are you working there? Remember that leaders are people who get others to perform at consistently high standards – voluntarily. If people do not enjoy their work, or feel valued, all the mission statements, quality circles, and team building exercises in the world will not achieve high performance.

Interestingly, Moss Kanter's 'F' words relate to the characteristics of organizations who have successfully coped with major change. Such organizations understand the importance of leadership, which means they are probably full of passionate people who dream dreams, have visions, and get other people to help them achieve goals. That sounds like fun.

In case you are wondering, the other 'F words' defined by Moss Kanter are 'fire' (as in, sacking people), 'fragility', 'façade', 'fear' and 'feudal'. (Alimo-Metcalfe 1993)

Effective leaders trust. Those paragons, effective leaders, also trust people to do a good job. We all know that trust is the bedrock of stable relationships, that if we do not have trust in each other then we spend time checking up on performance, meddling in people's work, and generally being miserable and cynical. But misery is optional. So is delegation, which is trust in action. Leaders love to give their followers room to hang themselves, because they know better than we do that we will *not*. Never tell a leader 'I could not possibly do that job', because they are sure to ask why, and then leave you to prove yourself wrong.

Delegation becomes a trial when we do not do it appropriately. Real delegation is not buck-passing, but is a crucial part of personal development. Leaders understand this, because they have a flexible view of how people work. A leader uses your potential, not your job description, to decide how much to delegate to you, and when. They watch you to praise and appraise (the checking bit), the aim being to help you move your performance to a higher level.

Effective leaders have values. Leaders live by their values. Values are our lodestar. Even if we go off course, they guide us to a safe harbour.

Without values, our decisions are made for convenience, and not to map out the appropriate way ahead. There are many examples of leaders who have paid the ultimate price for holding to their values. Some have lost their homes, their families, their jobs and their friends. You do not have to do anything dramatic to have your values tested. Something as simple as saying 'no' when others say 'yes, for a quiet life' is enough to test the strength of your values. We will return to the issue of values when we consider leadership for the 21st century, in Chapter 12.

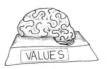

Effective leaders have passion. This is the heart of leadership. If there is no passion, there is unlikely to be commitment or drive for achievement. Think about what drives you, how much time you spend on it, how much you resent having to stop and do something else. To put it another way, if what you give is what you get, give it all you've got.

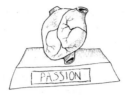

Passion is another one of those 'dirty words' that many organizations, including the NHS, loathe. Imagine, all those messy emotions, people wanting to share their thoughts and feelings, wanting to know what you really think and feel. Terribly sorry, we do not do that here.

I do not understand that attitude. We get out of our warm beds every day, leave our warm homes and families, sometimes travel miles to work, do our job in often dismal surroundings, miss lunch, work late, get ulcers, migraines, repetitive strain injuries and varicose veins – and have no passion for what we are doing? Maybe that is why we get ulcers, and the rest. Call me a fool, but if it lacks passion, work is not working.

Effective leaders are passionate about many things – people's capacity to learn, collaboration and partnerships, honesty, openness, and integrity. To put it simply, leaders seem to fall in love with what they are doing. Their enthusiasm rubs off on others, and everyone gets the chance to have their dreams addressed.

The sad part is we probably all start out passionate about what we do at work. But gradually the procedures, policies, imposed limits, and creeping apathy reduce passion to grumbling about the smallest thing. What distinguishes effective leaders is the way they *regenerate* their passion.

As you develop as a leader, never make the mistake of believing that you have to do a course before you can tackle a problem. In the same way that you cannot learn to ride a bike by reading about it, leadership has to be practised, and with a passion to achieve.

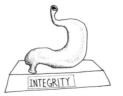

Effective leaders have integrity. Integrity can be defined as moral and intellectual honesty. There is an old saying, which goes: 'If you do not stand for something, you will fall for anything'. Such is the fate of the leader without integrity. Without integrity, leaders betray themselves and the people who follow them. Everything they do is for expediency, convenience, and short-term gain.

Think about some of the debacles that have featured in the media in recent years, and which have demonstrated most eloquently what happens when integrity is lost – MPs taking cash to ask questions in the House of Commons, a chief constable refusing to resign after criticism of serious flaws in an investigation concerning the death of a child, the sale of arms from the USA to terrorists in return for hostages.

Of course, having integrity can also get you into trouble. Think of the pathologist who was sacked because he 'blew the whistle' on colleagues for falsifying research results, and of Graham Pink, the nurse who was eventually dismissed form his position as a night duty charge nurse because he refused to tolerate poor conditions for his patients, and spoke out. I am not saying that leaders should respond to every criticism by throwing in the towel, and nor am I saying that leaders who retain their integrity are going to have an easy ride. But those leaders who are clear in their own minds about the standards of behaviour they expect of themselves rarely find themselves in a position that demands their resignation.

Sometimes I feel that acting with integrity is seen as old fashioned. But without it we will surely become even more cynical.

Effective leaders have political awareness. Successful leaders are politically aware and have really sharp political skills. The grid shown in Table 5.1 outlines four types of political behaviour commonly exhibited in organizations. Each part of the grid contains some of the characteristics of the behaviour. As you will see, leaders need to be politically aware, and be able to act with integrity. It is a myth that the two behaviours are incompatible, and that successful leaders bend the rules.

Women have a particular aversion to politics at work. In an article in *Working Woman* in 1993, Susan M. Barbieri puts it like this: 'Women tend to have extreme views of office politics. When they don't regard the game as one of ruthless backstabbing, they see it as a quest to collect best friends with whom they can share their secrets. Share no secrets, make no best friends. The office is not a pyjama party' (Barbieri 1993). Although I hesitate to agree with the 'no best friends' part of that statement, I feel Susan Barbieri is right. We go to work to get things done, to make life better for our patients. Liking the people we work with is a bonus. Our political antennae must be well attuned to opportunities to build alliances, communicate effectively, and help colleagues to do their job better.

It is no use being clever politically if people end up being damaged by weakness in the leader's profile in other areas. No leader can be truly successful for long if she or he is not trusted, or loses credibility through dis-

Table 5.1   The politics grid

Politically aware		Politically unaware	
Clever (psychological game-playing)	**Wise** (acting with integrity)	**Inept** (psychological game-playing)	**Innocent** (acting with integrity)
Knows how the formal and informal organization works Thinks before speaking Aggression masked by charm Insecure, but well defended Always leaves the job before mistakes are discovered Manipulative, appears never to make mistakes Good at playing power games	Knows what's on the grapevine Tactful and emotionally literate Checks information and rumour Loyal Open and sharing Can cope with criticism and being disliked Can see links between disparate issues Knows own purpose Knows the formal and informal organization Knows how to build alliances Knows who can, and who cares Skilled at negotiating and listening	Hates to be ignored Emotionally illiterate Unethical Does not understand politics Unable to make alliances Does not listen to others Sees issues as either/or, us/them Tends to speak in clichés	Believes being right = power Great capacity for friendship Has exaggerated respect for authority and rationality Tends to rely on authority Does not appreciate politics Loyal Sticks to the rules Sharing and open Equates authority with power
May say: 'I think it may be unwise for me to act … you are better at it' 'I have already discussed it very thoroughly and everyone agrees' 'I share some of those feelings, if not so passionately'	Likely to say: 'I wonder what lies behind that decision?' 'Let's look and see how we can get over this difficulty' 'Let me make sure that I haven't misunderstood you'	Likely to say: 'Let's decide what we want and make it look like it's what they want' 'We all know how she got her job'	Likely to say: 'In my professional opinion …' 'Can we stick to the main task of the meeting' 'If only they would tell me what to do, I could get on with it'

honesty. But on the other hand, there is little virtue in political innocence, no matter how much integrity is displayed. Leaders need to be politically astute, otherwise they may fail to build the alliances and networks they need to achieve their goals.

Effective leaders have a productive life position. Life position is a concept adopted from transactional analysis, and is the theme of Thomas Harris' book *I'm OK, You're OK* (Harris 1973). You might have heard the concept also referred to as 'Windows on the World' in which people talk about the 'frames' through which they view life.

Life position refers to the core attitudes and beliefs that we hold about ourselves and others, and about life itself. We use attitudes and beliefs to try and make sense of other people's behaviour toward us, but we often forget that the way we behave towards others affects how they respond to us.

Let me give you an example. Sally, a freelance trainer, is very sure that she can tell which people on any of her courses will be shy, and which will be more talkative. The basis for her claim? – the colour of their hair. People with red(dish) hair say almost nothing throughout the whole day, while those with black or brown hair are much more participative and talkative. However, if you saw Sally in action you would notice that, from the start of the course, she talks most to people with black and brown hair, and they respond in kind. She has few conversations, or eye contact, with participants with red hair and seems uncomfortable in their presence.

You can imagine some of the longterm results of Sally's beliefs and consequent attitudes. If you keep in mind that behaviour is beliefs and values in action, you will understand how a life position based on negative assumptions about yourself and others can impact on relationships.

There are four life positions, or frames, and these are summarized in Figure 5.2.

The four positions represent permutations of whether we think others are OK and we are not, or vice versa, or we are all OK or not OK. We can also consider it in terms of lose/lose, win/win, and all the other permutations.

Most of us will recognize that position (4) is one of mutual respect, acceptance and collaboration. In this position, we accept that we may have to compromise to get most of what we want and give the other person most of what she or he wants. But then there are those days when the world, from our point of view, conspires to mug us. On these off days, we tend to slide into one of the other, less productive, distorted, positions. Leaders also have off days, but they have the ability to stay focused on productive behaviours. I believe that they manage to do this by using proactive language, being open about their distress, and taking responsibility (that is, being response-able) for that distress.

Many of us assume that if it goes wrong it is our fault, and if it goes right,

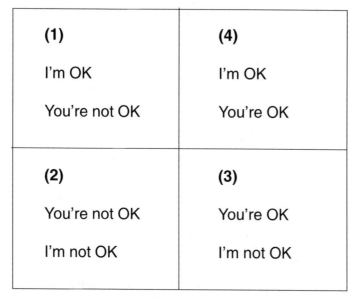

(1) I'm OK You're not OK	(4) I'm OK You're OK
(2) You're not OK I'm not OK	(3) You're OK I'm not OK

Figure 5.2   Life positions (adapted from Hay 1996, with permission).

we did it by ourselves. Such distorted attitudes are grounded in childhood experiences of being vulnerable, small, and helpless. Box 5.3 offers a few examples of how appropriate childhood life positions can become established features of our behaviour as adults. I will use the abbreviations for the life positions as in Julie Hay's book (Hay 1996), for example, 'I'm OK, You're OK' (IOKYOK).

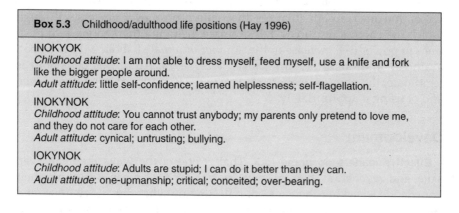

Box 5.3   Childhood/adulthood life positions (Hay 1996)

INOKYOK
Childhood attitude: I am not able to dress myself, feed myself, use a knife and fork like the bigger people around.
Adult attitude: little self-confidence; learned helplessness; self-flagellation.

INOKYNOK
Childhood attitude: You cannot trust anybody; my parents only pretend to love me, and they do not care for each other.
Adult attitude: cynical; untrusting; bullying.

IOKYNOK
Childhood attitude: Adults are stupid; I can do it better than they can.
Adult attitude: one-upmanship; critical; conceited; over-bearing.

Hopefully, in reading this book on leadership you are firmly in position (4). You may find yourself, however, straying into one of the distorted positions. That is OK, as long as you notice it, work out why, and move on. That is what leaders do.

Effective leaders use power. Leaders have a great regard for power. As with politics, they use power as a tool to assist in decision-making, goal-setting, and implementation (I prefer to use the word 'tool' instead of 'resource', which carries notions of being finite; on the other hand, as we assemble a set of tools, we become more skilled and expert, and more adept at adapting the tools).

Most books on power carry a list of the sources of power. Box 5.4 presents such a list, including sources not always mentioned in the books.

Box 5.4   Sources of power

- Organizational position
- Money
- Physical force
- Knowledge or expertise
- Social class, gender, race
- Symbols, such as physical space (desk size, designated car parking space, sole use of a secretary, size of office, hours of working)
- Personal power, or influence
- Language
- Tradition
- Physical resource
- Occupational group
- Social culture
- Alliances

While leaders may access these sources of power, and more, they focus on personal power and building alliances. Alliances are key to understanding why some people seem to be able to create their resources seemingly out of thin air. Through alliances, they gain control over processes through which they access resources. For example, helping others to get into positions of power (the increase in the number of female Labour MPs is a good example), and doing favours *without being asked*. All of this behaviour is legitimate; the point is, leaders recognize the importance of having power, and of using it appropriately.

Development

Effective leaders do homework. That is one of the ways they can keep sane, and regenerate their passion. By homework I mean refreshing their knowledge, checking their vision, reflecting on what they have done, and challenging themselves to be the best. I do not mean reinventing something akin to a school timetable.

In a video I saw some years ago, Tom Peters tells of visiting a friend's home for dinner. After dinner, his friend's father, a distinguished surgeon, excused himself, saying that he had to do homework for an operation he was performing the next day. Peters was surprised. After all, this doctor was respected, experienced and skilled. What more did he have to learn? 'It is because I do homework that I keep my skills', he answered.

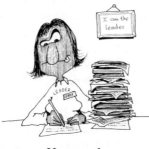

Homework

A leader's homework takes many forms – reading, writing, watching television, going to the theatre and the movies, listening to music, silence, talking, being with families and friends, or just staring into space. While writing this book, I rediscovered the power of meditation, the fun of browsing through books, reading as a pleasure activity, silence, and the joy that is dictionaries. My passion for developing people, and for writing, now has a new energy. The major beneficiary of doing my homework is me, because that is what goes into my work with people, and into my writing. Leaders who remain committed and passionate never pass up the time to do homework.

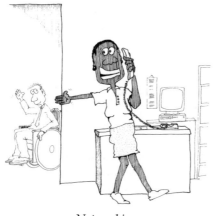

Networking

Effective leaders network. I will have to tread carefully here, because whenever I mention 'networks', I am often accused of wanting to 'perpetuate élitist models of development'. Until I find out exactly what that phrase means, I will continue to argue, passionately, that to maintain our personal and professional effectiveness, we must tap into a variety of sources of knowledge, contacts and information, including gossip (yes, gossip, which is a much underrated source of information and learning).

Networks exist, and can make the difference between success and failure. Let me give you an example. A few years ago, I organized a 3-day professional visit to New York for 40 NHS women managers. Because of the short time they would be in the city, I wanted them to meet with as many key people as possible. I telephoned someone I had met in New York while on a research fellowship, and simply asked him to suggest names of people I could call. Within 2 weeks, he called back to say that he had arranged a welcome meeting at the British High Commission, a visit to a famous hospital in Harlem, and an evening function with a former mayor of New York.

I had so underestimated the power of my networks, I was stunned. The visit was a huge success, and many other networks were established because of it. Several years later, this one event is about to spawn another network in a completely new area.

There are five types of networks:

1. Personal – friends, family, colleagues.
2. Professional – inside and outside the organization, if you work in one. If not, those associated with your work.
3. Organizational networks.
4. Strategic networks – organizations or people who share similar goals.
5. International networks, which can encompass the preceding four.

Leaders understand the power of networks, and use them appropriately. Networking is a key element in the process of continuous learning. They understand the value of knowing who is doing what, where, when, and with what result.

In Meredith Belbin's work on teams, one of the identified roles is Resource Investigator. These people are natural networkers, bringing back to their team news from the outside world. They illustrate in leadership terms what Picasso said about artists: 'Good artists copy. Great artists steal'. Leaders understand this, and are not ashamed of stealing good ideas, developing them, and *sharing the glory*. Leaders never forget to be grateful. Neither do they forget that networking is often more about giving than about getting; a common misunderstanding of networks is to see them as sources of personal gain, rather than as opportunities to enable others.

Not all networks are worth joining. Leaders are therefore highly discriminatory about how they network, with whom, and for what purpose. A leader's reputation is a great asset, and she or he would be unwilling to sacrifice it under any circumstances. When they network, they use the same approach they bring to other initiatives in which they become involved – consistently, systematically, and with crap detectors on full alert. This also means that leaders cull their networks when necessary. As with everything else, networks have a sell-by date. The key is to remain curious about what is happening around you, and develop the ability to use that knowledge to enhance your skills as a leader.

OVER TO YOU

If you have read the preceding section in one go, take a break. When you feel ready, tackle this next section, which gives you an opportunity to explore your development needs as a leader. There are five activities:

1. Life position analysis
2. Networking
3. The power questionnaire
4. Homework, or continuous learning
5. The environmental audit.

Activity 5 consists of a checklist to help you identify gaps in the support you need to develop as a leader, Activities 1, 2 and 4 consist of a series of questions or scenarios and Activity 3 is a self-completion questionnaire. It is not compulsory to do these exercises, or to show the results to anyone. However, listen to your thoughts as you decide for or against.

Activity 1 – Life position

The first part of this activity asks you to consider how much time you think you spend in each of the 'windows' (see Fig. 5.3). The easiest way to do this is to think of a typical day or week and reflect on the moments when you adopted each of the positions.

For the second part of this activity, consider the following questions:

1. What unsatisfactory interactions occur when I view the world from a distorted position?
2. What problems arise at work, and in my life, because of the beliefs and attitudes I hold about myself and others?
3. What do I fear most about giving up distorted behaviours?
4. What opportunities do I have for viewing the world from the IOKYOK position, even when under stress?
5. Who among my colleagues, friends and family are likely to respond positively to such a change?
6. In what situations can I feel safe to practise my new behaviour?

7. How will I know when I have learned to view the world mainly from the IOKYOK life position?

Activity 2 – Networking

Make a list of your networks using the following headings:

- Personal
- Professional
- Strategic
- Organizational
- International.

When you have done this, choose one of the headings and turn it into a mind map (see Fig. 5.3). Note the connections between the different people in the network. Are the same people in your networks? If so, are you limiting your networks to people with whom you feel comfortable? If all your networks involve circulating around the same people, think about expanding your horizons reciprocally and altruistically. You may find the following points useful in developing your networks.

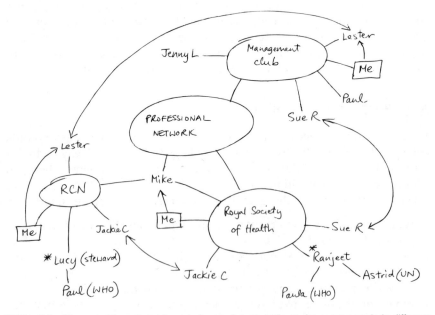

Figure 5.3 Example of a networking mind map. Arrows indicate the same people in different professional networks with whom there may be a tendency to associate with more than with others. In this example, note that more systematic and reciprocal association with Lucy and Ranjeet (starred) would be helpful as they have international contacts which would enhance the network.

Eight steps to rejuvenate your networks

1. Make a set of personal business cards. Many mainline rail stations have machines where you design your own cards. It takes about 20 minutes from beginning to end. The longest part of the process is waiting for the cards to be printed – so take something to sit on!

2. At conferences, give your cards to people you find interesting, and ask for theirs. On the back write the date, the event, and what you found interesting about them.

3. Staying with conferences, if you hear or read an interesting presentation but don't get to meet the speaker, telephone and let her or him know how much you valued what he or she had to say. Usually, the speaker will be surprised and pleased by your call (conference presenters do not get as many positive strokes as you would think – we assume that someone else will do that, so we will not have to. Anyway, we might be afraid of being taken for creeps. Which life position is this!?).

4. Spend one half day each month catching up on the gossip in your personal network.

5. Subscribe to the Internet and get an e-mail address.

6. Bluff your way into events/conferences to which you have not been invited. This is easier if you follow steps 1–3 above. Name-dropping has its (positive) uses.

7. Develop a range of interests outside of your profession. This makes you interesting, and a source of information for others.

8. Cull your networks – draw three circles (see Fig. 5.4 for example). In the inner one put the names of the people you talk to or see every day. In the next circle, the names of people you talk to or see one to three times monthly. In the last circle, put the names of those people you see or talk to twice each year or less. Every 3 months or so, review the circles. If your networks are helping your development, you will find that the names in the circles will change as people move closer or further away from you. For example, some of the people in the inner circle may move to the second circle, or may be removed altogether. Someone from the outermost circle may move into your inner circle. These changes must happen to some extent, otherwise your networks will stagnate.

Activity 3 – The power questionnaire

The focus of this self-completion questionnaire is your attitude to, and beliefs about, power. There are 10 questions, with four potential answers to each – A, B, C, and D. Circle one answer option for each question. When you have finished the questionnaire, total the numbers of As, Bs, Cs, and Ds. The scoring is on two fronts: power mode, and life position. The relationship between these two concepts is given in Table 5.2.

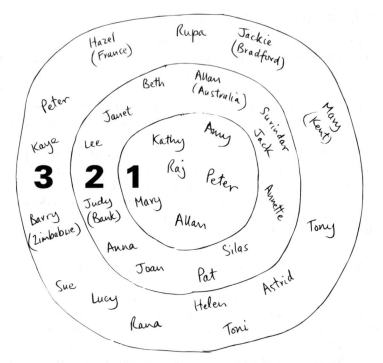

Figure 5.4 Example of diagram for reviewing networks (1) Daily contact (2) Monthly contact (3) Yearly contact. Note that there tends to be more people in (1) than in (2) or (3).

Table 5.2 Power mode and life position scoring

Power mode	Life position
Control freak	IOKYNOK
Brown mouse	INOKYOK
Balancer	IOKYOK
Pessimist	INOKYNOK

The Power Questionnaire (Drummond 1992)

1. The best method for creating power is to:

   (a) Have absolute control over everything.

   (b) Have influence and responsibility only in your area of work, as defined by your job description.

   (c) Have control over a few key issues.

   (d) Prevent others from getting your share.

2. A representative from a firm of 'head hunters' calls and wants to talk to you about a job you have always wanted. You:

   (a) Let them know they are talking to the obvious person for the job.

   (b) Say no.

   (c) Ask to see more details before you decide.

   (d) Decline as this is clearly a hoax phone call.

3. Your line manager is on long term sick-leave caused by stress. You:

   (a) Immediately take over her duties, as you are more competent anyway.

   (b) Wait until you are asked to deputize.

   (c) Agree to deputize, and tell your manager that you are happy to keep her informed of what is happening in the office in her absence.

   (d) Stand back and watch your rivals fight over who will deputize.

4. You want to increase your power in the organization. If you had a free day, how would you spend it?

   (a) Give your colleagues a detailed agenda of the day you will be spending shadowing a well-known chief executive in a private sector company.

   (b) You do not want a free day.

   (c) Attend a conference or drop in on colleagues in other departments.

   (d) Make sure the day is not counted as part of your annual leave.

5. You are an invited speaker at a prestigious international conference. You want to make a good impression, but you tend to stammer when under stress. Therefore, you:

   (a) Repeatedly tell the organizers that you will not accept requests to simplify your overhead projections. This only causes you stress.

   (b) Decline the invitation.

   (c) Use a tape recorder when rehearsing your presentation and practise not stammering.

   (d) Plan to tell you audience that you are nervous so they will not laught too much at you.

6. You are attending an important staff meeting, but you have not had time to read all the necessary papers. You:

   (a) Blame the internal post system for not delivering the papers on time.

   (b) Do not attend because you will look a fool for not knowing the answers.

   (c) Confess and ask the appropriate people to summarize the key papers you have not read.

   (d) Go to the meeting because nobody pays any attention to the meeting papers.

7. A colleague of long standing, who is also a friend, has received a promotion to chief executive. Do you:

   (a) Tell him all the bad points about his personality he has to change.

   (b) Decline his invitation to be part of his support group.

   (c) Congratulate him openly and tell anyone who will listen how good he is.

   (d) Watch to see how long before he drops you as a friend.

8. Someone has taken credit for something you have done. You:

   (a) Are surprised. You did not think they had that much intelligence.

   (b) Say nothing, but cry a lot.

   (c) Believe imitation is the highest form of flattery, but openly take revenge.

   (d) Expect nothing better.

9. You notice that a new member of staff looks unhappy, and not sure how to do their job. You:

   (a) Tell the person exactly what they are doing wrong.

   (b) Are surprised because they are more senior to you.

   (c) Befriend them and help them to settle in.

   (d) Ignore them – everyone here is miserable.

10. What colour would you wear to an important interview?

    (a) Anything that will shake up the panel.

    (b) Ask someone to choose for you.

    (c) Whatever is appropriate to that company, and what you feel comfortable in.

    (d) I am not stupid enough to fall for this question.

Scoring

Mainly As – *Power mode: control freak. Life Position: IOKYNOK.*
To you, power is primarily about things, and people, being the way you want them. This may be fine in some instances (such as in emergencies). In the long term, however, your relationships will suffer as people avoid what they see as attempts to manipulate them. You also lose because you fail to learn from others as you have a tendency to believe that you always know best (what one colleague called the 'fallacy of infallibility'). If you are seething while reading this, I will not take it personally.

Mainly Bs – *Power mode: brown mouse. Life Position: INOKYOK.*
You are likely to have problems with the whole concept of power. Much of the time situations overwhelm you, and you do not believe that you can

influence anything or anyone. The people who live and work with you may eventually come to resent your dependency, and your seeming inability to stand up for yourself (unless you are teamed with control freaks. But then they will criticize you ad nauseum). In the long term you may become totally unable to make even simple decisions for yourself.

Mainly Cs – *Power mode: the balancer. Life Position: IOKYOK.*
You have a healthy regard for power, understand its uses and limitations, and are unlikely to worry if things do not go as you planned. You are not afraid to reveal your real feelings, while remembering that others are not as advanced in this respect as you are. In the long term, your attitudes toward power and your productive Life Position may irritate others who take a more jaundiced view of life. But then, you know this already(?).

Mainly Ds – *Power mode: pessimist. Life Position: INOKYNOK.*
My mother always said that a pessimist is an informed optimist. So there is hope – if you balance the cynicism with a little humour. You are painfully aware of the power of power. You probably read Nicolo Machiavelli's *The Prince* and recognized in it everybody with whom you work. You are right to question people's motives, but only up to the point when they are proved to be suspect. Many of us are up to no good at some time in our life, but we do not deserve to be pre-judged before and after the event. In the long term, your power mode and Life Position may jeopardize personal and work relationships.

If you really aspire to improve as a leader, the best power mode and life position to strive for is balancer and IOKYOK. The others are distorted views of how the world is. This is not to say that people do not have ulterior motives. You can look through the IOKYOK window and make honest judgments about what is really happening, not make it up to suit whatever play you are writing in your head.

ACTIVITY 4 – HOMEWORK

This is a simple activity. You may want to use the results from the Power Questionnaire to devise a development plan which may include reading some of the books listed at the end of this chapter. At the very least, devise a timetable to include some or all of the following, plus whatever else you may be doing:

- Day-dream.
- Read your professional journal.
- Start (or continue to develop) your portfolio and personal development plan.
- Get nosy through your networks.

- Take an evening class in a subject that interests you. Learning is a transferable skill which is best based on topics of interest.
- If you need to, take an accredited course of study.
- Read science fiction, general fiction, unknown authors.
- Generally, understand that life is not school. We have several chances to learn how to do better.

ACTIVITY 5 – THE ENVIRONMENTAL AUDIT

Box 5.4 is a checklist of the factors that support the development of leaders. Depending on what support you need, you may decide to weight each factor according to its importance to you. If your organization has a leadership development programme, you may want to see if these support systems are in place.

Box 5.4 Factors that support the development of leaders

- Potential leaders are openly supported and developed
- Mentoring schemes
- Peer learning-sets
- Mistakes are welcomed
- Financial support processes for accredited programmes (for example, refunding 50% of fees paid, or all the fee if a certain grade attained)
- Senior managers behave like leaders
- Skill inventories (for example assessment centres) to support personal development plans
- Opportunities for development available to everyone, regardless of position
- Senior managers take lunch breaks away from their desks
- Vacations are sacrosanct (that is, people take them)
- The organization works with and supports local voluntary groups
- The chief executive is not called 'Chief Executive'
- Celebrations and laughter are routine
- IOKYOK is the predominant Life Position.

Key learning points

- Effective leaders see the world as it really is

- Distorted Life Positions can lead to distorted interpretations of our own and other people's behaviour

- Politics and power are legitimate pursuits

- Effective leaders understand the need to network and do homework

- If you need support, ask.

FINALLY, SOME TIPS ON GETTING SUPPORT

Ask.

REFERENCES

Alimo-Metcalfe B 1993 The F words. Health Service Journal, July: 25
Barbieri S 1993 Office politics in the nicer '90s. Working Women August: 34–37
Berne E 1968 Games people play. Penguin, London
Covey S R 1999 The 7 habits of highly effective people. Simon and Schuster, London,
    pp 81–85
Drummond H 1992 Power: creating it, using it. Kogan Page, London
Harris T 1973 I'm OK, you're OK. Pan, London
Hay J 1996 Transactional analysis for trainers. Sherwood Publishing, Watford

11 things you might not know about effective leaders

1. Leaders do not walk on water 91
2. Leaders take lots of holidays 92
3. Leaders are made of rubber (resilience) 93
4. Leaders do not always win 94
5. Leaders are politically astute and even wise 95
6. Leaders have active crap detectors 95
7. Effective leaders are generally emotionally stable 96
8. Effective leaders are not always the most intelligent 97
9. Effective leaders stick to their objectives like glue 98
10. Leaders like to hug and be hugged 99
11. Leaders often do not know that they are leaders 100

Key words:

emotional stability; politics; crap detector

At this point in our analysis, it might be useful if you took a little time (about 10 minutes) to write down any myths you have heard about leaders.

The list of 11 things that you might not know about leaders include their weakness for fun, hugs, and holidays. I have collected this list over many years and experience of working with many leaders. Some of the things on the list have been researched and can be found in text books (for example, emotional stability, resilience); others, like the crap detector, are features I have observed and been intrigued by. As you examine the list, check your own, and reflect on your own behaviour as a leader and the experience you have had of being the led.

1. LEADERS DO NOT WALK ON WATER

Otherwise known as aquatic perambulation, walking on water is one skill that many leaders may acquire due to over-attention to hubris. This activity is often driven by an unfounded belief in the omnipotence of the leader, backed up by the conviction that they can do what they want, when they want, with few negative consequences. Previous success has clouded their judgment. The circle of people who give such leaders advice prefer to tell them what they want to hear. Reality is not allowed to interfere with a chosen action. Remember that consistently effective and successful leaders have their feet firmly on the ground, although their heads are sometimes in the clouds. Leaders who harbour a belief in their ability to walk on water are usually in need of the kind of dispassionate advice they are unlikely to seek. Let me give an example.

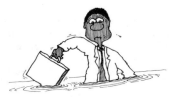

Leaders do not walk on water

In the early days of the 1991 reforms of the health service, a colleague who managed an acute hospital was adamant that the changes would be totally beneficial. There was no cause for concern – money would follow patients to whatever providers they attended. Hospitals would be more efficient and staff who had reservations were simply unwilling to take risks, and poor at adapting to change.

This colleague had had a successful career, and had won the admiration of most of the people who worked for him. He was bright, personable, and good at his job. He expected his future to be as bright as his present. So committed was he to the reforms, that it became impossible to have a conversation with him if you expressed doubts about the process. Gradually, I stopped calling him for a chat.

About 18 months into the reforms I happened to hear a radio discussion about the NHS. Managers were expressing despair and frustration about the changes. One of the most despairing was my colleague, who was incensed that the reality was turning out to be so different from the publicity. His inability to fully assess what was happening in the here-and-now affected his capacity to lead. He failed to assess the future and was left disillusioned, with very wet feet. At least he did not drown.

If you know any leaders who have this habit, notice if they have webbed feet. If not, do not copy them.

2. LEADERS TAKE LOTS OF HOLIDAYS

Some of the failings of organizations can be traced to tired people – people who do not take enough holidays. I know that the tendency is to judge commitment to the job by how many hours you work in any one week. But ask yourself: what do I do in 60 hours that cannot be done in 35 or less?

And if the answer is 'we have no staff', ask all your colleagues the question: do patients really benefit from being cared for by people who are tired, irritable, and over-worked?

When I worked as a senior manager in an RHA, I would insist that staff took all their holidays, and that they took their lunch break every day unless unavoidable. I also recommended that they spent the first day back at work from holidays catching up on gossip. One of the highest compliments ever paid to me was that I had an innate streak of laziness. I took that to mean that I do not do things for the sake of activity, and that I know when to stop, look, and listen. If anything derogatory was meant, I refused to take offence, and comforted myself with the knowledge that some of the greatest discoveries came during times of relaxation and reflection.

Real holidays give time for repose, lazing, idle staring, dreaming, and doing the kind of things that recharge the batteries. 'Working holidays' are not in this category. All work and no play not only makes us dull, it also keeps us from knowing ourselves, our friends, and our families. I find it very strange that people will seek counselling to manage stress, but never think of reducing the things that cause the stress in the first place.

Because effective leaders know they are indispensable, they happily go on holiday, and forget the office. An example of this is the man who once managed Avis Rent-a-Car. Robert Townsend would go off on holiday and not tell anyone when he was coming back. He would simply send a memo to say which of his assistants would be in charge during his absence. When he returned, he took no reports of what had gone on in his absence. As far as he was concerned, the person he had left in charge was competent to do the job – no report necessary. You might find it useful to read Townsend's: *Up the Organization*, and *Further Up the Organization*, in which he talks about leadership, organizations, and people (Townsend 1977, Townsend 1988).

Some leaders take holidays from their regular job to do something in which they have a passionate interest. Some go back to study, change careers (one highly-regarded city banker reportedly left his job to enter the priesthood), or take up a hobby. Because these changes in direction are usually planned, and are committed to, issues that worry you and me – mortgages, paying the bills – are equally well managed. Which brings me to the next thing. The resilience of leaders.

3. LEADERS ARE MADE OF RUBBER (RESILIENCE)

The *Concise Oxford Dictionary* defines rubber as a 'tough elastic polymeric substance'. Rubber is used to erase pencil and ink marks. I cannot think of a more fitting substance for effective leaders to wrap themselves in. Remember the stories in Chapter 2? Those six people had the bounceability of rubber. That is probably just as well, given the tenacity you need to meet some goals. They make it seem so effortless, but every effective leader I have known seems to have a fine seam of steel running through their rubber coating.

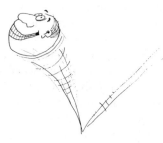

Leaders are made of rubber

The rubbery nature of leaders gives them resilience, but rubber can corrode. This does not mean they never fail, or never have doubts, or never want to give in. They just never give up, but keep bouncing back, probably indefinitely.

4. LEADERS DO NOT ALWAYS WIN

I breathe a sigh of relief whenever I hear about leaders who have setbacks, just like mere mortals. But, wait a minute. It is not their fault if we choose to think they are not mortal. We are simply perpetuating a myth. Leaders fail, get it wrong, disappoint their followers, and generally mess up. They are made of rubber, not Teflon. And bad things can happen to them. A colleague of mine lost her job because she would not make reductions in infection control services, reductions she knew would cause a deterioration in the infection rates in her unit. About 2 years after she left, her predictions proved accurate. The rate of wound infections increased by about 5%, anaesthetists began demanding that used intravenous cannulae be once more randomly sent for microbiological examination, and the head of the surgical directorate had to review the infection control policies.

If leaders always won, they would be insufferable. But *we* are the ones who load them with the mask of invincibility. Truly great leaders are as likely to talk as much about their failures as their successes. They do not, however, make a virtue of losing. Losing is just another chance to learn what not to do, and how not to do it. So, do not feel that you have to offer sympathy – it will be accepted, but not expected. Instead, ask for a front seat when this person starts to dissect how she or he fouled up.

One of the most educative and entertaining afternoons I have ever spent was in the company of three women who, leaders all, swapped stories of their worst leader-in-crisis moments and, even better, shared how they had learned to accept their failings without weakening their resolve. That may be a hard lesson for you to learn, but think of the consequences of not learning that lesson – forever being afraid not to win, afraid to fail. A ward sister once said to me that she did not mind if I made mistakes, as long as I did not make the same mistake twice, in the same way. That is a lesson that many leaders learn the hard way. If the lessons are internalized, that is probably due to fact number 5 …

5. LEADERS ARE POLITICALLY ASTUTE AND EVEN WISE

I know I have talked about this at length in Chapter 5, but I make no apology for repeating myself. Being politically skilled and politically aware is a key attribute of effective leaders. But nurses still persist in ignoring the politics of the organizations they work in – and not just nurses. Most people who work in organizations shy away from politics. Like a dirty secret, politics is shoved to the back of the consciousness.

If you have this attitude, please give it up. Politics is the grease that makes the cogs turn. At its simplest, politics concerns a set of beliefs and principles which govern our actions. In an organization, politics concerns authority, status and power. We cannot avoid politics, because it exists however much we want to ignore it. Effective leaders are good at politics, meaning they are good at making alliances, using their influence, and knowing how organizations (that is, people) tick. If you are still ambivalent about the role of politics in creating effective leadership, go back to the *political awareness* section in Chapter 5 (pp. 74–76), and also look again at your response to the corresponding self-evaluation.

6. LEADERS HAVE ACTIVE CRAP DETECTORS

Would you follow anyone who led you into danger because they took the wrong advice from the wrong person? Of course not. This is where the crap detector comes in.

I first read about the crap detector in a book written for newly-qualified teachers. The concept appealed to me, because it rang true. The crap detector works like this: from every ten pieces of information you hear, eight are useless. Of the remaining two, only one is of any real value, the other being just padding.

Crap detecting is about deciding what to keep, and what to jettison. One way I have found that works well is to note from whom the information is coming. A friend? An enemy? A potential ally? To make this easier to see, look at the diagram in Figure 6.1, which I call the Survival Matrix.

Can you see how important it is to be able to categorize your informant? Can you also see how easy it is to confuse opposition with enmity, and fellow-travellers with new converts? It is a common enough mistake, and every leader makes it at one time or another. Caught in the intensity of pressure to act, our judgment may be clouded. The crap detector must therefore be kept on at all times. If you are clear about your purpose, actively listen to and reflect on what is said to you, it will be much easier to sort the wheat from the chaff.

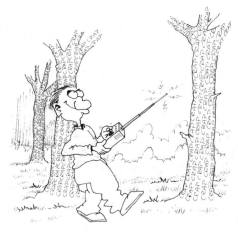

Crap detecting

Using this matrix has helped me on several occasions, especially when I was getting information overload. By using the matrix, I have generally managed to reduce my information sources to the tried and tested, the ones who have proved accurate and relevant over a period of time. This does not mean ignoring other sources, it simply means being wary until proven otherwise.

7. EFFECTIVE LEADERS ARE GENERALLY EMOTIONALLY STABLE

For the past 2 years, there has been much press attention to something called 'emotional IQ'. Put simply, people with a high emotional IQ are nicer to have around. They are less likely to have poor, dysfunctional relationships with others, and are more likely to add value to the job they do and the people they work with.

Emotional IQ is probably a leadership-theory-in-the-making. It makes perfect sense for leaders to like people, and we all like to work with nice people who are stable, who take a balanced view of events, and who are not easily put off by disappointment. People who have these qualities are far more likely to be effective. Emotional stability in a leader inspires self-esteem and self-confidence, and makes it easier to get things done.

Allies	Opponents
Allies are people who believe in what you do and support you; they also watch your back; they may be friends.	*Opponents* are allies who do not agree with a particular action that you are taking.
Bedfellows	**Enemies**
Bedfellows are people who hitch their wagon to your star, as long as you are going up; they are opportunists.	*Enemies* are people who dislike everything you stand for; they may try to harm you; they do not like you.

Figure 6.1　Survival Matrix. I first came across this during a lecture given by Rennie Fitchie.

Emotional stability also implies a realistic approach to meeting objectives, the ability to laugh at oneself, and a refusal to take oneself seriously. Emotional stability also depends on stable, healthy relationships with family and friends, although this doesn't necessarily mean that all relationships run smoothly, or exist in a rosy haze. Effective leaders get their fair share of personal trauma. They just gather their emotional resources to handle it better. Leaders who spend too little time building these personal support systems of friends, family and play will only be effective in the short term. And a high intellectual IQ is not a substitute.

8. EFFECTIVE LEADERS ARE NOT ALWAYS THE MOST INTELLIGENT

Do you remember the Great Man theory of leadership outlined in Chapter 3? One of the characteristics of this person was that he would be the most intelligent in any group of which he was a member. Proponents of this theory believed that high intelligence was the mark of a great leader. But research by Meredith Belbin on how groups work produced surprising results. Highly intelligent people put in a group and given an objective performed poorly, because they spent their time fighting to get their own ideas accepted by the whole group.

From this work, Belbin developed the now famous Belbin Team Roles, of which there are 8 (Belbin, 1981). The roles are based on personality types and levels of IQ. One of the roles is that of Chairman, who has the task of ensuring that the group remembers, and meets, their purpose. On the Belbin scale, the roles with the highest IQ scores are Plant (PL), and Monitor Evaluator (ME). Having facilitated numerous groups, I met only one PL in a leadership role, which he hated, and one ME, who had some difficulty with interpersonal relationships.

High IQ does not mean effective leadership. It can mean impatience with others who are slow off the mark, arrogance, and poor work relationships. Some of the most effective leaders I have worked with used techniques such as Belbin Team Roles to identify the strengths and deficits in their group, and therefore knew how to use people's skills to the optimum.

9. EFFECTIVE LEADERS STICK TO THEIR OBJECTIVES LIKE GLUE

Do you know someone who goes on and on about one thing until you want to scream? Sorry, you have just met an effective-leader-in-the-making. These people quite simply have the bit between their teeth and nothing, short of dynamite, can shift their focus. Before you finish nodding in agreement, there is a caveat. They can be shifted, as long as that means refining the goal, not giving it up.

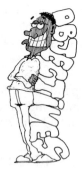

Effective leaders stick to their objectives like glue

The issue might be simple, like how the telephone in reception is answered. They know it can be done better, we know it can be done better. The difference is, a leader will act to make it better. Hence the almost continuous questions (often beginning with 'Why?'), the probing, and the monitoring. Eventually, for a quiet life, you give in, and find that it is always easier to ride a horse in the direction in which it is going – meaning that a leader committed to changing or maintaining something for the better is not easily driven off course. Eventually, you will appreciate this tenacity, because they do not give up on people either.

One of the buzz statements in many organizations is that 'our staff is our greatest asset'. Senior managers also stress that they want people to take initiative and risks. But all the fine words are likely to melt away should we make a mistake. I have painful memories of hearing the reason why, in one hospital, midwives did not hold babies while they were bottle feeding, and propped the infant up in a cot instead. Several years before, a midwife had dropped a baby, and since that time they had been forbidden to hold babies when feeding them.

Apart from denying a newborn baby the comfort of human contact, the practice was dangerous. The babies would toss about, and the midwives would have to hold the babies' heads to maintain a steady flow of milk. Babies do not like having their head held, especially during the first 12 hours after birth. Stroked yes, clutched – no. It probably will not surprise you to learn that in that particular unit, staff were far from happy, and mothers often complained about the quality of care they received.

We really cannot except people to follow us as leaders if we give up on them at the first false step. Effective leaders are most supportive when their followers are faltering.

10. LEADERS LIKE TO HUG AND BE HUGGED

At the risk of causing misunderstandings, let me clarify this. Every successful and effective leader I have known has been a people-person. I don't mean this in the 'touchy-feely' sense; I mean that they value human relationships, and are emotionally attached to what they are doing. One result is a willingness to give and receive affection.

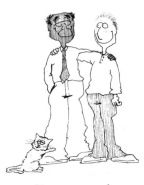

Hugs are good

No, this stuff is not imported from the USA. We all need literal and figurative hugs. Leaders give and get hugs in abundance. This makes sense. Would you follow someone who was emotionally distant, who was uncomfortable with talking about your feelings about what you do, and became nervous if you expressed doubts about your ability to meet agreed objectives? As a leader, would you expect anyone to follow you if you had these tendencies?

I once had a book called *The Little Book of Hugs*. If I remember correctly, it gave all kinds of excuses for hugging – success, tears, happiness, just for the hell of it. If mass-endorsed, that book would probably be of more benefit to the gross national product than any number of technological advances. You do not have to terrorize people, or force your attentions on them. But physical contact, appropriately applied, can work wonders.

Effective leaders know this, and do it brilliantly. One of my first experiences of this was with a night sister when I was a student nurse. She was a former nun and she hugged you with her voice. She was so focused on enabling students that you felt better just by being in the same room as her. Another ward sister had the happy habit of yelling 'God bless and safe journey home' to all staff at the end of every shift. None of this was done for effect, and neither of these women would have called what they were doing a part of leadership.

11. LEADERS OFTEN DO NOT KNOW THAT THEY ARE LEADERS

A long-standing custom in the health service is that we do not share good practice, and therefore do not learn from each other. In 1997, I had the privilege of being a judge for the National *Nursing Times*/3M Awards which, each year, recognize excellence in nursing practice. I was awed by the entries. The variety of approaches to leading change was striking. Making visits to short-listed entrants was even more overwhelming. There were no fancy offices, no frills. Just solid leadership driving caring practices.

What I found particularly striking was the surprise that some entrants expressed at being short-listed. This may be cultural – British reserve, and hiding lights under bushels. But this cannot be the only explanation. Many of us have bought the idea that leadership is the province of those who are at the top of the hierarchy. We may be doing brilliant work to improve patient care, but do not make the connection with leadership. We assume that because the need to change is so obvious to us, it must be to everyone else. If you think like that, you are becoming a leader.

Remember Aaron Feuerstein in Chapter 2? He did not know why some people were so surprised when he decided to keep his staff on full pay while the burnt-out factory was rebuilt. After all, he believed that superior staff gave superior service, so should be treated in a superior way. It was very simple – to him. But to others?

Now you can understand why leaders need to be emotionally stable, resilient, and have crap detectors. Without these, they would probably leave us and go and live on another planet. Leaders do not *do* leadership, they *lead* – by example, by action, and by believing that they can make a differences. If you spent your time *doing* leadership, you might get to know a lot about the theory, and rarely get a chance to practise. Leaders just *do* it.

Let us reflect on what we have talked about. Leaders and leadership have been surrounded by so many myths that is difficult to sort fact from fiction. Many of us look to others to provide leadership, believing that we cannot do it ourselves because we have not been touched by some higher power. We seem to want our leaders to be both omnipotent, and human. We castigate them when they fail to live up to these unrealistic expectations, while reserving our right not to become leaders.

We cannot have it all ways. We cannot honestly expect others to take on tasks that we are not prepared to perform ourselves, to make decisions we are not prepared to tackle. We cannot expect our chosen leaders to take responsibility for our uncertainties and our fears. Leaders are only as good as their followers. If nurses are to thrive, we have to step out, step up, and accept our potential as leaders. That means having a clearer idea about how leaders behave, what they do, and how they survive.

A starting point is to be more realistic about the whole concept of leadership. A friend once said that the more you talk about a thing, the less energy there is to do it. Leaders think *and* do. This might explain why many effective leaders seem puzzled by our reactions to what, to them, is the obvious. It might also explain why we sometimes find them so hard to live with. To leaders, it is simple – if there appears to be a problem, identify it, and fix it if it needs fixing. If complaining is a solution, then do it to optimal effect. If not, do not bother. Even people in positions of leadership, however, forget this simple approach from time to time.

Remember the chief executives who expressed frustration at not being able to influence healthcare policy? I want to quote from the article in the *Health Service Journal* which reported on the forum in which these views were expressed: 'Some participants looked enviously at the policy influence wielded by groups such as the Association of Chief Police Officers and the Association of Directors of Social Services, and the formal establishment of a continuing organization for chief executives was considered … The proposal [to set up an organization] was eventually rejected in favour of organizing two more forums next year, under the auspices of the chief executive's development programme' (Butler 1997).

Yet some in the group felt that chief executives 'should be prepared to take more risks where constructive criticism of government was needed'. I am sure that the decision to wait was arrived at after much debate. But what if this new programme, untried and untested, left the chief executives as frustrated as before? They would have lost a whole year of possible action, while two existing models, *which were envied for their success*, were rejected.

It would be interesting to know whether the chief executives who wanted to form a continuing organization, and not just meet in a forum, were more frustrated at their position than those who wanted to wait for the new programme. Not being privy to the whole discussion of the first forum, I hesitate to say that the decision to wait was wrong. But a year is a long time, and the frustrations are not likely to go away, whichever government is in power.

What will the chief executives do in the meantime? Yes, they will go to work, but how effective can you really be if you feel paralyzed by some events, and believe that others have power over your decisions? How will this affect the people who look to you for leadership? Do they know how you feel? If they do, does this mean that they will screen their conversations with you, and not tell you about *their* frustrations? If they do not know how you feel, might they see your decisions as inconsistent and woolly, and cause an increase in your frustrations?

This is just the kind of self-questioning in which effective leaders engage. They know that every action on their part has an effect on others, and vice versa. Sometimes this might lead them to appear to be overly slow and cautious in taking action. But if you were climbing a mountain roped to a leader, which would you prefer: one who had planned for known risks, and had taken advice about possible risks from the whole group, or one who went off half-cocked? Whether mountain-climbing or in more mundane pursuits, having an outline answer to such questions could save your life.

You may want to follow the process of the chief executives' forum, because their deliberations are likely to be covered by the *Health Service Journal* and other periodicals. On the other hand, you may want to ask your own chief executive if she or he shares the same frustrations of not being able to influence policy, and if that is likely to change. Reflect on how the

Key learning points

- Among other things, effective leaders are politically skilled, resilient, emotionally stable, and have active crap detectors.

- Becoming a leader does not require saintliness.

- Leaders give in, but never give up, especially on people.

things leaders do in your organization affect how you perform – and vice versa. Because you are not a saint, angel, or perfect, neither are leaders. Part of becoming an effective leader is learning what you do not know about yourself, but your followers do.

REFERENCES

Belbin M 1981 Management teams. Butterworth Heinemann, Oxford
Butler P 1997 It's tough at the top. Health Service Journal, 6 November: 12–13
Townsend R 1977 Up the organization. Coronet, London
Townsend R 1988 Further up the organization. Harper Business, London

7

The trouble with leaders

Key words:

unique; aliens; envy; sex appeal; life positions

In the last chapter, we dismantled some of the myths about effective leaders. To square the circle, let us spend some time considering some of the things leaders do not know about themselves.

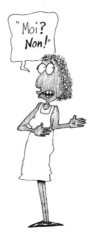

No, that can't be me?!

The selection of observations that are presented in Box 7.1 are not scientifically tested. They are tendencies I have noticed in all the leaders I have met, worked with, and talked to.

> **Box 7.1** Leaders' tendencies
>
> - What leaders do is unique
> - Leaders are few in number
> - Leaders are scary people who make some of us nervous
> - Leaders are from outer space
> - Leaders are sexy
>
> - People would do (almost) anything for them
> - Leaders have one-track minds
> - They are terrible to live with
> - We envy them

UNIQUE BUT NOT THE ONLY ONE

First, what effective leaders do is unique. I do not mean that leaders are unique as people, or that the work they do is unique. I believe that we are all potential leaders, when circumstances demand. Their uniqueness is in how effective leaders *lead*.

The key words are 'consistent', 'systematic' and 'forward-looking'. Remember that leadership is about getting consistently high levels of performance from people, without coercion, bribery, covert persuasion, or other forms of control. This makes sense. Can you imagine getting people to give high quality work consistently by using any of these tactics?

Effective leaders also work systematically, or deliberately, if you prefer that word. Actually, 'deliberately' is a better word, because it describes exactly how effective leaders do things – intentionally, purposefully. It also echoes a phrase I like to use when coaching – 'be on purpose'. Effective leaders do not have projects without a plan, or teams without a clear purpose. Being systematic (or deliberate) does not necessarily mean being boring, nitpicking or overly cautious. It does mean taking time to think through what needs to be done, exploring possible ways of doing it, and taking account of obvious consequences. Being systematic (deliberate) is part of respecting other people, their time and their energy levels.

Like Alison introducing Tea Tree Oil for mouth care (Chapter 2), the ideas for change that leaders get may result from serendipity, but from then on, the way the change is handled is purposeful. Effective leaders frequently ask themselves what I call the 'Monday morning at nine o'clock question': what must I do first, otherwise nothing else can be achieved? This is indicative of a systematic, purposeful approach to activity, and links to the third key word, 'forward-looking'.

Spending time looking forward is part of day-dreaming. You can tell when someone is day-dreaming. She or he will have this slightly vacant look, and may be smiling gently, if not inanely. Some leaders I have worked with get this look, but when the day-dream ends, they will have formed some plan of action. Effective leaders are 'on purpose' when they day-dream. And they don't call it day-dreaming, but 'thinking about how it could be when ...'

Many of the leaders I know would not claim that what they do is unique. As far as they are concerned, it is just common sense to fix something if it needs to be fixed. Neither do these leaders spend much time analyzing their every action. They tend to see everything they do as leading to their goal, so their job and their life's work are closely intertwined. This conjunction might take time to develop and reveal itself. The development path is one of transformation, from 'what I do', to 'how I do it', to 'how did I come to be doing this?' In Chapter 9, we will look in greater depth at transformational leadership. For now, let's just think about a leader's transformation, from doing tasks to questioning the motive behind their actions, as being part of their uniqueness and of their search for better things to do.

A SCARCE COMMODITY

Which brings me to the second thing that leaders do not know about themselves – they are few in number. A few years ago, I heard a well-known nurse say that nursing has many leaders, but no leadership. I have since come to understand that the use of the word 'leaders' in this sense invariably refers to the positions people hold, and not to the leadership function – getting people to perform at consistently high levels, voluntarily.

I do not mean to sound trite, but there are few leaders because few leaders meet the definition above. Leadership is still misconstrued as being associated with rank and (usually senior) position within the organization, with followers being those at lower levels – whether they choose to follow or not. That this is a nonsense is becoming clearer, even to the health service. After all, if you continue to believe that leadership is a position and not, as Kouzes and Posner so elegantly put it, 'a performing art' (Kouzes & Posner 1995), what is the point of talking about self-managed teams, teamworking, and cross-functional working?

Being few in number, leaders are in great demand. You know the expression 'if you want something done, give it to a busy person'? Leaders have destructive demands placed on them, because people know they will deliver. The problem is, *they* do not believe they are few in number. They might suggest we contact some other person whom they regard as a leader, and who may even be their role model. No, we say, we do not want any others, only you – please come and help us. I remember once turning down a job because I discovered that nursing practice developments would be put on ice until I arrived to sort it all out. I ran for my life. While I gladly accept challenges, and have as one of my aims lasting innovation in nursing practice, I had visions of that job turning into a burden, and not a shared experience with colleagues.

Making unreal demands creates unreal expectations, which leads to disappointment, blame and victimization. Worse, we often expect our leaders to read our minds and find (by osmosis?) what we want them to do. When they do not meet our unspoken needs, we get upset, sulky, and nasty. Leaders who fall into this trap end up having to play 'rescuer' to our 'victim'. If we give them enough hassle, they may even become our 'persecutor'. In organizations, many failures of leadership follow this pattern, which follows the rules of a well-known game in transactional analysis called 'yes, but ...' Look at the following as an example of the 'yes, but ...' game in operation.

Leo is a nurse manager with a high profile in his field. An opportunity arises for him to be seconded to a unit similar to his own, where he will be responsible for implementing a change in nursing practice. A similar change was attempted a few years ago, but failed when the change agent did not get on with the staff.

Leo has many ideas of how the change can be implemented within a given time and with limited resources. But each time he suggests a plan of action to deal with staff's concerns, he is given any number of 'yes, buts ...' For example:

- It cannot work here.
- We tried that before and it didn't work.
- They wouldn't let us do that.
- It will cost too much money.
- We don't know how to do that.

In exasperation, Leo asks why they have bothered to invite him to come to them if they do not really want to change. The staff then feel even worse than before they started, and the game goes on.

Many people in organizations play variations of this game. Leaders who fall into such traps that we (knowingly, or unknowingly) set for them, can easily become blocks to their goals.

SCARY STUFF

It is probably human nature that we sometimes fear that which we desire most. Over the past 2 decades at least, we have yearned for leaders who will protect us, heal us, and generally make us feel better. Using past experience as a guide, however, most of us believe that the price tag for such rescue missions is too high – dictatorship, coercion, manipulation, erosion of civil liberties.

If only we could find nice, friendly leaders who did not demand too much of us, who did not remind us too often of the commitments we have broken, who would collude a little with us. What do we get instead? A bunch of people who actually do what they say they will do, who talk out of turn, and who speak the truth as they see it. Who do they think they are, frightening us with all this talk of 'accountability', 'responsibility', 'ethics' and 'standards? Don't we have enough to worry us?

When we say we want leaders with integrity, honesty, morals and humour, leaders take us at our word. They do their best to challenge our complacency, our failure to do what we know is right, and our cowardice. They do not give up on us, they do not blame or victimize us, they do not lead us where they will not go themselves. In their mind, we have set them a challenge. Their aim is to get us to volunteer in meeting the challenge, which we do with varying degrees of commitment and energy. All they ask for is our best, but sometimes being our best seems too much effort.

Many of the leaders you and I know would probably not agree that they are scary people who make others nervous. But I wonder if deep down, some of them scare themselves? When you act purposefully and get results, it can seem that you have a special pact with some force beyond yourself. On the other hand, it may just be that, unlike the rest of us, you have a clear idea of what you want to do, set up a plan, and execute it. Simple? Yes – and scary. Because many of us have no plan, no aim, no clear purpose.

If you think this is a harsh judgment, ask yourself this question: if you were guaranteed success in anything you did, what would you spend the rest of your life doing? I have asked several dozens of people this question. The majority respond that there is no guarantee of success in anything. Actual and potential leaders consider the question and answer along the lines of 'what I am doing now, and maybe something else, or better'. The concept of guaranteed success (or not) does not seem to faze leaders. They are so focused on doing well in what they are doing now, and scanning the future for opportunities to do better things, that the intensity of their commitment guarantees a result of some kind.

Leaders know that rewards come from commitment. The greater the commitment, the greater the reward. Success, of some kind, is therefore guaranteed. It all depends on how you measure success and against whom you measure yourself.

The scariness of leaders is precisely this quality of having different benchmarks against which they measure their performance. While many of us are probably content with doing what is expected of us, leaders are doing what is not expected – going that little bit further. This 'surprise' factor is probably the most unsettling habit of leaders, and it does make us nervous. But remember, leaders are not endowed with super powers; they are ordinary people who do extraordinary things. If they can do it, why not us?

Because they are not like us.

ALIENS

Leaders are from outer space. They must be. That is the only logical explanation I can think of to explain their weirdness. By outer space I do not necessarily mean from another universe. I mean that they seem to inhabit another dimension where integrity, commitment, magnanimity, creativity, dedication and humility are accepted and acceptable currencies. Where people speak truthfully, no matter how unpleasant it may sound. Where consistency and constancy, not conformity, rule. A place where principles is not the name of a clothing store, but things by which people live and act.

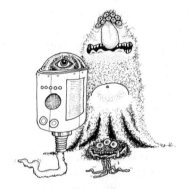

Leaders from outer space

A spot check of the people who live in this 'other dimension' would reveal the following odd behaviours (well, odd by 'normal' standards):

- Not taking sides
- Not sweating about the small stuff
- Spending an inordinate amount of time talking about their work, not who they are
- Never using the word 'failure' (instead talking about mistakes, missteps, errors of judgment, accidents)
- Liking people
- Maybe being eccentric, but not neurotic
- Eating anything, at least once
- Not judging people
- Liking their own company
- Having a passion for living.

Not all of them have all of these quirks to the same degree. But if you speak to one of them, you can bet your last 50 pence that somewhere in the conversation you will begin to get the strangest sensation that the person in front of you is not From Here. Her dress may be familiar, but she talks a different language.

Go back to the exercise on life positions you did in Chapter 5. To save you time, Figure 5.2 is reproduced again here as Figure 7.1.

Remember that most of us try to live most of the time in section (4) – we feel good about ourselves and other people, we act assertively as appropri-

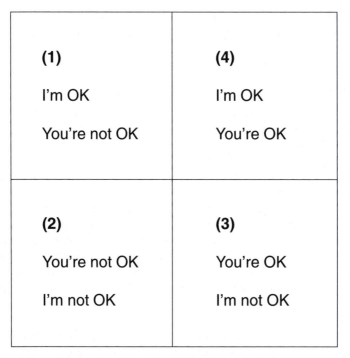

Figure 7.1   Life positions (adapted from Hay 1996, with permission).

ate, and are generally productive. When we become stressed, however, we tend to revert to the other sections. We all have a greater or lesser tendency to live out one or more of the destructive life positions. What are your tendencies?

People from the Other Dimension rarely leave the life position in section (4). That is probably why they exasperate us, always seeing the positive in every circumstance, not unlike Jane Bennett in *Pride and Prejudice* – but with a slight twist. They don't wear rose-coloured spectacles. Leaders are head and heart, thought and action, poets and warriors. The world they inhabit is multi-dimensional, where every problem has some kind of solution, and everyone has something to offer in solving the problem.

To some of us, the weirdest thing about leaders is that they believe they are normal. They believe it is perfectly normal to have goals and dreams, share them, refine them, and make them happen. Leaders have little trouble with living in outer space because it is just another version of the present, and anyway, they are having fun. We also long to be as weirdly normal as them, but without the hassle of the 'vision thing', and the 'commitment thing', and the 'consistency thing'. In the next chapter, when we look at why leaders fail, and fail to lead, I will come back to this weirdness that I have noticed in leaders. For now, hold on to the idea that people who exhibit weirdness invade our imagination, and undoubtedly have a certain sex appeal.

SEX APPEAL

In the context of leadership, 'sexy' is more about behaviour than physical attraction. I do not mean that some leaders are not physically appealing. But the nature of a leader's sexiness is closely connected to how she or he treats others and responds to their ideas. It is associated with their general lack of self-absorption, their interest in you as a person and what you are capable of achieving.

All this can be seductive, especially if you are accustomed to not having your feelings, ideas and opinions respected. Who would not find even moderately attractive someone who, when speaking with you, gives you her or his whole attention, treats your ideas with respect, and *listens* as well as hearing what you have to say? Usually, this interest in you is not feigned, and stems from the clear motive of helping you help them to achieve their goal.

Admittedly, some leaders have manipulated others in pursuit of their own ends. Such behaviour tends to lead to failure, as we will see in the next chapter. Effective leaders may feign interest in many things, but their fundamental respect for people prevents them from using coercive tactics to get your attention.

Effective leaders are also sexy because they are committed to something, and are willing to act to achieve their aim. Link this to their lack of self-absorption, and you have a basic recipe for charm. Add a dollop of success, a dash of ego and an ounce of old-fashioned good manners, and many of us would be willing to walk a few extra miles for this person. The icing is power, which is very sexy. And effective leaders are powerful people.

Remember that having a 2000 watt personality is not a necessary requirement for effective leadership. Most leaders do not have overwhelming personalities. But that does not mean they are not powerful. They make things happen, they get people to act voluntarily, they inspire, they are purposeful. All this adds up to considerable *personal* power. If a leader also has positional power (that which comes with a job), she or he has an added advantage. But it is personal power that enables leaders to achieve their goals successfully, and which makes them attractive to people.

It is fair to say that most effective leaders, even the shy ones, would admit that they are powerful. We are all attracted to power, and like to be around powerful people.

CLOSE TO YOU

You probably know at least one person for whom you would stop doing whatever you were doing to assist them if they asked. Effective leaders can have such an impact on our lives that people have been known to walk through fire (literally) for them. Such behaviour has little to do with brown-nosing, and everything to do with the consequences of leadership.

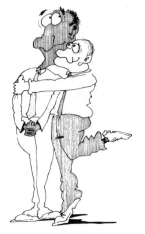

Anything for you, my leader!

We would do almost anything for effective leaders because we know they would do the same for us. Going the extra mile for a leader whom we respect and trust is more than just a function of the job in hand; it grows from the human relationships between leaders and followers. In Game Theory there is a concept called *reciprocal altruism*, or Tit for Tat (Axelrod 1984). Put simply, if on first asking you cooperate with me, I will use the result of this as the basis for all further interactions with you. This is exactly what leaders do when they share their visions and refine them in the light of comments from others. By initiating cooperation, they are more than likely to get a similar response in return.

We know it works, because we do it every time someone asks us for a 'favour'. We know it works because we talk about people who 'do right' by us, or who 'are there for us'. We do not work well with people who take, and give little in return; who are uncooperative, under-handed, and generally out for themselves.

MONOMANIACS WITH VISION

The prominent management guru Peter Drucker once said that if in an organization you find something happening, look for a monomaniac with a vision (Drucker 1988). I prefer the term 'committed to the future'. It sounds less pejorative, but means the same thing – total attention to the job in hand, including getting the resources to achieve the goal.

Being a monomaniac with vision may strike you as an exhausting way to live. But leaders and their volunteers (or followers) thrive on this commitment to their goals. I do not meant that they subordinate their lives to one issue – some do, with varying degrees of personal trauma. I *do* mean that leaders are focused, purposeful and action-oriented. They may take several years to achieve their goal, but they do not lose sight of what they want to do. The same applies to their volunteers. Let me give you an example by telling you a story I heard recently.

Maureen (not her real name) is a very talented chef. She was employed by a large organization in that capacity for 10 years, until she was dismissed. With no savings to speak of, she set out to achieve a lifelong ambition – owning her own catering business. Although people will always want to eat, catering is not the most stable of businesses to be in. Fads and fancies change, and contracts are often secured through word of mouth. But Maureen had her dream.

Using contacts she had made while an employee, she obtained small assignments at first. As her new customers told others of the quality of service she offered, her business grew. One of her biggest contracts now is with her former employer. Maureen employees up to 10 people, depending on the assignment, all of whom are former colleagues or friends. They get paid, but they work with her as volunteers, because she enabled them to dream their own dreams.

Maureen's one-track mind probably never contemplated working for someone else after her last employer. She worried about bills, mortgages and all the other things that cause us to hesitate to fulfil our dreams, but she marshalled her volunteers, shared her visions, saw the opportunities for success, and jumped.

Maureen denies that she is a leader, but she does 'admit' to being committed to what she is doing, and to helping others (especially women) live out their dreams. A one-track mind can take you on several journeys at once, as long as the direction is forward.

COME LIVE WITH ME

Such intensity of commitment can be stressful to live with. Not only do leaders day-dream purposefully, they also want to tell you all about it. It does not matter to them that you may have heard the same dream before (this is Day-Dream Mark 60), you must listen. They don't *force* you to listen – on the contrary, their enthusiasm for what they are doing is catching – but being contrary, we want the enthusiasm, not the consequences. If we share lives with enthusiastic, often restless people, a consequence is that it may rub off on us.

The trouble with leaders is that they cannot stop wanting things to be different. Their restlessness can cause those with whom they share their lives great concern. Florence Nightingale's parents had nightmares about her future. Anne Smith's student colleagues probably tensed every time she opened her mouth. Alison Mennie's colleagues say jokingly, 'What will you get up to next?' It can seem as if leaders already live in the future and bring us news from there on a daily basis. But many leaders would probably be horrified at the suggestion that they do not live in the present. As they see it, they focus on the future and that is why they can live in the present. They would say that looking forward gives them the strength to plan, act and change. If they could not perceive a future of better things to do, and to do some things better, they probably would not bother getting up in the morning – until they had a found a solution to that particular problem.

This is a state common to us all at some time, but knowing it may not help if you share any part of your life with effective leaders. At best, they are spell-binding; at worst, repetitive, mono-focused, and unapologetic about their enthusiasm. I am both fortunate and cursed to share my personal and work life with several effective leaders. There are days when I pray for no dreams, when I do not want to think about the future, and certainly do not want to talk about it. After about a day of this self-indulgence, however, I find I am missing the flights of fancy, the Jupiter-based thinking, and the buzz from being with people who have been caught by their own imagination. It would be terrible not having them in our lives. We envy them, even as we sometimes try to shield ourselves from their energy.

GREEN-EYED MONSTERS

I am often asked to speak to groups of women about 'how to be successful and effective'. The first few times, I was very flattered. After that, I started taking these requests very seriously. Instead of talking about me, I asked groups to explore their own meanings of success, and what they would be willing to pay to achieve it.

This format worked well for several such meetings, until I presented a workshop on personal effectiveness to a group of midwives. About 5 minutes after I began to speak I became aware of the hostile body language of three of the participants – tapping feet, almost glaring at me, and generally waiting for the chance to contradict everything that was said in the group. One person saw her chance when the topic was opened for in-depth discussion. Her question was: 'Do you have any children?'

I had answered 'no' before it struck me that the real question had not been asked. Deep breath from me, and I plunged in with: 'What does having children have to do with success?' By bits, the debate opened up into how women in the group used, and accepted, *organizational* definitions of success – which has meant that women with children are greatly disadvantaged in terms of promotion. I, being childless, therefore had no trouble in 'making it' in large, hierarchical organizations. After all, 'it's all right for you, you don't have any responsibilities'.

If you define success as promotion within an organization, and you believe that you are prevented from achieving this success, then envy of those who do climb the hierarchical ladder may be the result. But we mask this in various ways, partly because there are strong social codes against displays of envy. We may envy leaders their power, their access to resources and networks, or their seeming omnipotence. We do not often stop to consider that, by spending our energy on envying what leaders do, we limit our own ability to lead in our own way. No two leaders think or act in exactly the same way. Neither do they succeed in the same ways. When we hold envious feelings about someone's capacity to achieve her or his goals, we become blind to what we can learn from her or him.

The leaders we envy would probably be surprised that we have such feelings towards them. After all, they are not getting in our way – we are. Remember the 'Yes, but ...' game above that Leo got caught in? Envy is similar. Consider a leader you envy, for whatever reason. If that person was to give you a blueprint of how she or he successfully achieved a goal, would that ensure your success with a similar issue? Unless we are going to clone, Dolly-like, whole sets of leaders, then we will have to accept that some people will succeed better at some things than at others.

If you do have feelings of envy about any leader you know or work with, you might want to re-read the section of life positions in Chapter 5 (pp. 76–78), and look again at the corresponding self-evaluation in the same chapter.

Key learning points

- Leaders are unique, but are not the only ones of their kind.
- Leaders adopt a win/win life position.
- Envying leaders means we cannot learn from them.
- Playing Tit for Tat makes a journey bearable.
- Leaders are aliens with a one-track mind who are hell to live with.
- We love the leaders who love us.

REFERENCES

Axelrod R 1984 The evolution of cooperation. Basic Books, New York
Drucker P 1988 Management: the tasks, the responsibilities, the practices. Butterworth Heinemann, Oxford
Kouzes J, Posner B 1995 The leadership challenge: how to keep getting extraordinary things done in organizations. Jossey-Bass, San Francisco
Hay J 1996 Transactional analysis for trainers. Sherwood Publishing, Watford

Why leaders fail

Key words:

hubris; learning to learn; blind-spots and group think; Warren Bennis

There are no good leaders or bad leaders – just leaders who lead well or badly. So far we have looked mainly at the first type. It is now time to look at the flip side, what Jay Conger calls 'the dark side of leadership' (Conger 1990). I want to explore with you some of the reasons why leaders fail (as in, not learning from their mistakes), and to help you reflect sensitively on the flaws we all have which can create unnecessary problems for ourselves and others. Let me start with a story.

DEADLY DELUSION

Once upon a time, there were two schools of nursing, both with distinguished, if conventional, track records of nurse training. They saw themselves as rivals, competing for the same kind of student. Both curricula were heavily dominated by doctors, and little had been done to put more focus on nursing theory and practice.

There was little contact between the two sets of tutors, or even between the two hospitals who undertook nurse training, although they were situated less than a mile apart from each other. The poor contact was reflected in study days. Nurses from one hospital sat on one side of the room, nurses from the other hospital on the other. Group work never quite bridged the divide.

At the time our story begins, in the 1980s, education boards around the country were rationalizing schools of nursing (that is, reducing their numbers), and were developing the frameworks which would prepare nursing to become part of mainstream higher education. The two schools were geographically close, and offered almost identical programmes within the same small catchment area of the hospitals they served. This, and their medically-focused curricula, made them sitting ducks for rationalization.

The education board had reviewed both schools, and advised that they merge and substantially revise their curriculum, or both face closure. The time scale for completion was set as 1 year.

It is fair to say that the education board had previously advised both schools that their future was uncertain, especially with regard to the transfer of nurse education to universities (Project 2000 was in its first year). But it appeared that neither school had fully realized the implications of the education board's conclusions that they were not viable over the long term and needed to form local alliances with other schools, and with local universities and polytechnics. By the time they decided to act, it was already too late.

To add to the plot, general management was beginning to make inroads into the professional domain of nurses, doctors and other such groups. This was creating new demands for financial and other types of accountability. The two hospitals duplicated services, and each had a full complement of specialities, yet there was no visible attempt on the part of many of the senior managers of the schools to make the connection about the structure of their services, the changing nature of nursing practice, and the larger world of healthcare management.

I first became aware of the main issues when I attended a small meeting of tutors from both schools. It was clear that there was almost insurmountable resistance to the education board's warnings and predictions. There was also veiled hostility to my suggestion (I was new) that both schools should not take students for the next intake, but spend that year preparing to change. This would mean that the pre-Project 2000 student nurses could complete their training without having to compete with Project 2000 students, who would make significantly different demands on both tutorial and ward staff. Also, tutors would have some time to prepare themselves (and ward staff) for their first Project 2000 intake, and begin to learn with (and about) their colleagues from the 'rival' organization.

It was a tense meeting, the more so because the management structure of the schools was also being revised. Many nurse tutors didn't (and possibly still don't) accept that the new era of general management applied to their situation. A few weeks later, a full meeting of all tutors from both schools was tearful, with many recriminations. It is difficult to say precisely what effect all this had on the students of both schools, but many of the schools' managers seemed paralyzed, held hostage to their own assumptions about the nature of the changes which were influencing the direction of nurse education. Seemingly unable to shake off their own fears, their colleagues were mostly left alone to make their own adjustment to the coming changes.

Fear creates its own inertia, outside of which our old friend Chaos moves at will. Riding on the back of the proposed merger of the two schools, senior manager positions were also rationalized. One morning there were seven managers, and by the end of the day there were four. Some of these managers were as unprepared as their colleagues for the New World, holding to the belief that hospital managers could not possibly understand how nurse education worked, and could be made to see that a merger would not work. These beliefs prevented the creation of a 'shadow' senior managers' group to guide the merger, and to manage the new school in the first year. No plans, much pain.

The merger was messy, and the new organization had three heads in the space of 3 years, one of whom stayed for barely 10 months. The senior managers who survived the merger were the ones who had accepted the inevitability of change, and whose suggestions for turning the merger from a trauma into an opportunity were most likely to have received a brusque response from colleagues.

During the year when the two schools were facing the need to change, senior managers in both schools received lukewarm support for what they had to do. They in turn seemed unable to engage their colleagues in creating the best future for the new merged school. The majority of tutors in both groups spent more time fighting each other than facing reality. Both were caught up in their shared past as rivals, and could not see how they could be allies. The merged school also lost out on a key opportunity to join another as part of a university department. This second mishap revealed deeper problems – suspicions of people thought of as 'other', an unfounded belief that they could pick and choose allies, the apparent inability to learn from previous mistakes – but that is another story.

What this tale illustrates is a situation that occurs quite commonly in organizations: the inability of many leaders to read the environment with enough accuracy to prevent mishaps. Such leaders' need to maintain a distorted view of reality prevents them acknowledging that there is a problem. They are aided in this by followers who often would much rather have a nice, stable world than face the intrusions of a sometimes haphazard universe.

Of course, we followers would never consciously admit to such behaviour, but our unconscious selves prefer leaders who peddle us snake oil solutions to the fundamental challenges inherent in change, or any of the other issues that we would rather not face. We blame our leaders when the whole show goes southwest. We consider ourselves to be the innocent victims of venal politicians, rapacious businessmen (and a few women), and self-serving media robber barons. Unconsciously, we conspire to frustrate our leaders. This 'unconscious conspiracy' is the subject of a book by Warren Bennis, guru to gurus.

CONSPIRING AGAINST LEADERSHIP

Bennis' book is entitled *Why Leaders Can't Lead*, and its subtitle is *The Unconscious Conspiracy Continues* (Bennis 1989). Bennis has spent several years researching leadership and leaders, and being a leader. His book makes interesting reading for two reasons:

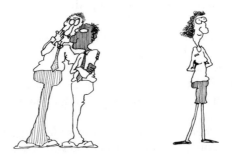

Do you know what she did the other day … ?

- It is an eyewitness account of leadership failure at the highest levels of public and corporate life.
- It places responsibility for the failure of leadership squarely on the shoulders of all of us.

Ouch. Bennis' argument is simple – not only have we, the people, let leaders down. We have also, through our systems of government, education, business, and self-absorption, actually conspired (unconsciously) to hamper any leader who wants to do things such as tell us the truth.

The running theme of the book, which is written from a US perspective, is the lack of heart and soul in organizations, and the general alienation of people from their work, their neighbours and their communities. From Bennis' point of view, the Superego (or conscience) has been upstaged by the Id (ambition). Everybody wants to be their own boss; competence (the ego) counts for little. In this Judge Dred-type landscape, people feel justified in creating enclaves of the like-minded, where 'The Other' is not allowed to intrude. The concept of community is lost, and we with it. To get out of this mess, conscience and competence have to retake centre stage from ambition. People, however, seem unwilling to give up the unreality in which they are living, preferring to opt for a simulacrum.

Now, if you have ever stayed in the USA long enough to pay rent (or watched enough episodes of any US sitcom), you will understand some of this. Wall to wall television, no need to leave your house to shop, to eat, or to be entertained. No need to mix with the Others if you do not want to. This insularity affects people in different ways – some become politicians and seem to make decisions based on the spoutings of the latest talk show host. Others lose the use of their limbs and are unable to communicate except by appearing on chat shows.

What makes Bennis' book so bleak is that the conditions under which the unconscious conspiracy thrives appear to be strengthening. Those conditions include:

- the substitution of hubris for vision
- the overwhelming focus on the 'bottom line' in business
- the increasing 'redundancy' of whole workforces
- apathy about politics and politicians
- a rise in crude nationalism and racialism
- disillusioned young people
- boredom.

If we look at our own country, we can see similarities. The advent of satellite and cable television and the wholesale importation of US ideas and cultures carry every possibility of creating a generation with short attention spans, wanting quick fixes to everything. To be fair, you do not have to be a 24-hour TV zombie to emulate our US cousins. Debates on the UK's place in Europe always remind me of a TéléFrance programme I saw in the 1970s. The reporter was gauging the feeling among a group of British teenagers about making learning a foreign language compulsory for school children. One young man was a model of Euroscepticism: 'Why do I have to learn French? I'll never live in France.'

Insularity is not new. Neither is our unwillingness to engage in an honest way with how the world really is. We are increasingly cynical about the calibre, motives, behaviour, and candour of our leaders. If it is not the 'fat cats' of industry who make us spit, it is government ministers involved in dubious activities, or funny-peculiar ways of awarding contracts in the NHS. Apart from grumbling down at the pub, or shouting at the television set, we seldom act to demand better.

But while I can agree with Bennis that we may unconsciously hinder our leaders, I do not agree that this prevents them from leading. Remember, leaders are made by circumstances, by accident even. This is not the same as being self-made, as in 'self-made woman'. There are many examples of self-made women and men who failed as leaders. Real leaders are made of burnished material – like humility, honesty, integrity, and an inability to consistently win popularity contests. They lead first, and follow when necessary.

The problems start when leaders begin to deliberately deny reality, my definition of Jay Conger's *Dark Side of Leadership* (Conger 1990).

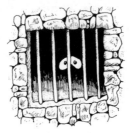

The dark side

LET THERE BE DARKNESS

Conger's focus is also the corporate world. He argues that the very characteristics that distinguish leaders from managers are the same ones which can harm the leaders and their organizations. Conger's examples of leaders who failed for one reason or another are all well-known public figures and visionary, charismatic leaders. All eventually failed at their task because they fell over their own feet.

Conger offers four reasons why visions fail:

1. The leader focuses on internal needs and neglects those of customers and others.
2. The leader miscalculates the resources needed to achieve the vision.
3. The leader has an unrealistic and distorted view of customers' needs (this is linked to the first failure).
4. The leader fails to redirect the vision in response to environmental changes.

If the leader remains blind to the fact that the vision is failing, even when her or his actions lead to negative results, then the really bad stuff begins – otherwise called 'cognitive dissonance'. You probably have your own examples of this, for example, the person who continues on a course of action to prevent damaging their positive perception of themselves. According to Conger, leaders who behave like this will use certain types of communication and impression management skills to keep reality at a safe distance. The potential liabilities of such behaviour include:

- Group-think.
- Idealization by 'yes' women and men who are dependent on the visionary leader.

- Use of anecdotes to distract from negative news.
- Creating illusions of control.

Conger's examples include John Delorean (who tried to create a new car company), Dr Edwin Land (inventor of the Polaroid camera), and Lee Iacocca, who ran the Chrysler car company (please do not read anything into the fact that all of Conger's examples are men; women leaders can also become victims of their own publicity, or general hubris. Margaret Thatcher and Indira Ghandi come immediately to mind). But in the NHS we have our own home-grown examples.

The NHS remains particularly vulnerable to large scale failures of leadership, partly because we are an insular bunch, and partly because macho management styles are still prevalent. For example, a report about financial mismanagement at Tayside Health Board talks of a 'secretive' and 'unprofessional' regime. One manager explained the board's misdeeds thus: 'I believed what happened was in part a result of the culture of the internal market' (Limb 1998). A similar defence was made in relation to financial irregularities within Yorkshire Regional Health Authority. Clearly, the internal market had the power to remove an innate sense of right and wrong.

One interpretation of what Bennis and Conger say is that the command-and-control leadership style of many organizations (plus the fractious nature of organizations in general) may predispose to failures of leaders and leadership. The command-and-control style concentrates power and patronage in a few people at the top of the organization. Remember in Chapter 3, we talked about transactional versus transformational styles of leadership? Transformational leaders are more likely to encourage participation and share information and power, and are less likely to develop the 'cult of personality' and group-think that can result from the 'one-man band' type of leader.

Interestingly, Bennis has lately begun to focus on the dynamics of groups, rather on leaders. In an interview with *Management Today* (Caulkin 1998), he said that great leaders only exist in a 'fertile relationship' with a great group. He calls these relationships 'creative alliances' in which both the leader and the group help each other to find their greatness. This is a near perfect description of transformational leadership, and women leaders, and those they lead, more often describe this as their style than do men leaders.

If you want to refresh your memory about these arguments, go back to Chapter 3 and review the section which summarizes Judy Rosener's and others' research into this issue. In Chapter 9, we will look at the growing need for transformational leaders.

The things that go wrong for leaders can be relatively simple, but it is how they react to hitches in their plans that matters. Let me illustrate this with another story.

BLINDLY LEADING

A few years ago, there was a 'little local difficulty' for a hospital manager who was investigating complaints by in-patients in a small specialist unit (part of a larger hospital) of ill-treatment by staff. The unit was in the process of being closed, and such allegations had been made previously, with no action being taken against staff. The current set of allegations, however, were more serious, and included complaints of victimization of patients.

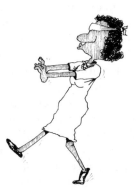

Blindly leading

A local patient advocacy group had challenged the way the closure was being handled and the manager's seeming lack of interest in the patients' complaints. The hospital manager in question had long experience in the NHS, was competent at his job, and thought that the advocacy group was stirring up trouble. It was not long before the local newspapers and community politicians were expressing their views, all in favour of the patients.

Relationships between the manager and the health authority, between patients' relatives and the managers, and between the hospital manager and the leader of the advocacy group, deteriorated and skidded out of control. A mediator was brought in to attempt to mend the relationship between the hospital manager and the leader of the advocacy group, and to bring some balance and objectivity to the issues. It quickly became clear that the manager had begun to see the problem as a personal attack on himself. It also became clear that the leader of the advocacy group was very politically astute, being careful to brief local politicians and the press when necessary.

The impasse between the manager and the advocacy group continued for several months, until the issue became a national news item. The manager exhibited signs of 'cognitive dissonance', seemingly unable to stop the behaviour that was producing such negative results. Eventually, he was 're-assigned', and later continued his career in healthcare management. An independent investigation into the specialist unit found some evidence of abuse by staff.

It is hard to understand how an intelligent person can be so blind to obvious flaws in his view of reality. According to Chris Argyris, however, smart people can find it difficult to learn. In what I think is one of the most important papers ever written on how adults learn, Argyris relates the story of a group of consultants who were debriefing their senior colleagues on why a project they designed had failed. The focus of the consultants' report was how unprepared and ill-equipped the client was. Until Argyris intervened to ask what impact they themselves had had on the project, the consultants and their senior colleagues had only looked at one side of the story (Argyris 1991).

This 'single-loop' learning is what stops smart people from learning. Unable to see how they interact with their environment, they expect the world to adapt to their version of 'how it should be'. To learn, a double-loop is needed. This is the bit that enables us to make a change in our behaviour, so that we do not make the same mistake twice, in the same way.

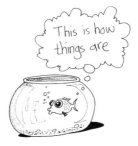

In a single loop

ADULTS AND LEARNING

I want to digress a little here and talk briefly about how adults learn. Reflect on the following quotation and its implications for personal effectiveness:

 We thought the trouble people have in learning new theories may not stem from the inherent difficulty of the new theories as from the existing theories people have that already determine practices. We call their operational theories of action *theories-in-use* [author's italics] to distinguish them from the espoused theories that are used to describe and justify behaviour. We wondered whether the difficulty in learning new theories of action is related to a disposition to protect the old theory-in-use. (Argyris & Schon, in Kolb 1974)

We have many opportunities for learning, but only when our behaviour changes can we say we have learnt. The quotation from Argyris and Schon sheds light on why many adults so often do not learn effectively from experience. We prefer the safety and comfort that the already known gives. We might say that we welcome new experiences, that change is a 'good thing'. We might even speak in favour of 'new brooms'. But scratch the surface, and you will find a strong veil protecting the current belief and behavioural system. We say one thing, and behave completely differently.

Take the example of the mantra, 'our staff are our greatest asset'. Yet we speak about *human resources* (resources are things that we use up and rarely replace), and spend peanuts on staff development, talent spotting and non-monetary reward systems. Eventually staff become cynical, especially when the training budget always takes the first hit when finances are tight.

I am sure that managers mean well when they say they are 'working toward equal opportunities', but the actual behaviour is often far removed from the espoused belief. To give up current beliefs and behaviours is to admit that all is not well. This admission creates vulnerability and invites self-criticism, which threatens self-perception. But the more we court safety, the less adaptable we become, and the more fixed in our views. We consequently have greater difficulty in accepting change, modifying behaviour, and in learning from new experiences.

The fear of failing, of not coping, of feeling incompetent, of being 'shown up,' are common responses to any event that seems threatening. Leaders who get caught in the 'single-loop learning' trap ultimately fail, not because they make errors of judgment, but because they fail to learn from the experience. The only time we can be sure that we have stopped learning is when we are dead. Until then, every experience carries the possibility of enhancing our capacity to be better leaders, and better volunteers of other leaders. (Of course, if you believe in reincarnation, you simply get to go round again and correct this life's errors. You hope.)

WHAT WOULD CAPTAIN PICARD DO?

When you examine your behaviour as a leader, what do you see? Do you, consciously or unconsciously, court 'single-loop' learning or 'double-loop' learning'? Do you hold on to a belief or idea even when the sell-by date is past? Do you accept that your plans are always subject to change? How do you respond to criticism, of any type? Are your decisions based on what you believe people will think of you, or on what you know to be right? What life position do you normally adopt?

These are some of the questions that might be asked of some of the health service leaders who have been implicated in high-profile failures over the past decade. While preparing this book, the events of the Bristol Royal Infirmary (BRI) painfully unravelled. My curiosity was roused by the apparent lack of nurse leadership for a group of such vulnerable patients as babies undergoing major surgery.

Some clues were given in the *Health Service Journal*'s report on Helen Stratton (Davidson 1998), the liaison sister in the paediatric cardiac surgery unit. Two small sections of this report seemed significant in terms of how leadership can be held hostage by an inability, or refusal, to accept reality. Helen Stratton suggested that a frightened teenage boy should go home because, in her judgment, his psychological state was too poor to cope with a serious operation he was to undergo. Accordingly, she consulted the chaplain, only for Mr Wisheart (the senior surgeon) to take her aside and tell her not to interfere with his clinical practice. The report then quotes Helen Stratton: 'Unless you have an understanding of how hospitals run, you don't know that it is impossible to go and knock on someone's door and say that something has to stop'.

Long before the tragic deaths began, leadership of the BRI seems to have failed at several levels – nursing, the board, medical staff, and directors. It is difficult to find another explanation for the apparent low regard for nurses in the hospital, the apparent failure of the chief executive to act on information about the poor performance of doctors, and the silence of nurses. The BRI case joins Kent, Exeter and Devon, Wessex, Yorkshire, the Blood Transfusion Service, Leeds General Infirmary, and South Thames on an inglorious list of major breakdowns of leadership in the health service. What I find alarming is the similarities in these failings – hubris (BRI, Wessex, South Thames), group-think among some senior managers (Yorkshire, South Thames, BRI, Blood Transfusion Service), poor standards (Kent, Exeter and Devon, Wessex, BRI) – and a general *laissez-faire* attitude to running a service. It is as if each part of the health service – health authority, hospital, GP practice, regional office, the centre – has become hermetically sealed from the others. Within these different parts, people also appear to be cut off from each other, so that common experiences are not shared or learnt from. Each error appears to be new to the environment in which it is occurring.

The philosopher George Santayana said that those who do not learn from their past are doomed to repeat it. Sometimes I feel that the health service repeats the same mistakes, in the same way, over and over again. It is just the degree of error that changes – usually upwards.

What do you want to do about this? How can we change this tape? Take a moment now to complete Exercise 8.1.

Exercise 8.1

Study the following pairs of sentences. From each pair tick the one that best matches your beliefs now. Mark an X against the one which you would like to be more associated with you.

1. Fearful of change.
   Excited and exhilarated by change.

2. I prefer to be with people I know.
   Strangers are future friends.

3. Not coping is a sign of incompetence.
   I do not have to do everything myself.

4. I never ask for favours.
   I need help.

5. People should be nice to each other.
   I need to learn to swim with barracudas.

6. People who resist change are not worth bothering with.
   Change is not always necessary, good, or beneficial.

7. If you are not my ally, you are my enemy.
   Disagreement is not the same as dislike.

8. Do not bring me bad news.
   Bad news = room for improvement.

9. Conflict makes a workplace unhappy.
   Principles are worth the loss of a job.

The first sentence of each pair carries a hope that the world will work according to how I believe it should. The second sentence of each pair is not the opposite of hope, but envisages the possibility that in every situation there is scope for both learning and improvement, even at a cost to ourselves. In a sense, one response to Bennis and Conger is to ask: how do we create the kind of leaders who will not succumb to conspiracies or the negative aspects of leadership?

A LEADERSHIP MOT

The next section of this chapter is a diagnostic exercise. The purpose is to help you spot flaws in your leadership style. The task is simple, and follows in Exercise 8.2.

Exercise 8.2

1. Do a self-diagnosis for each of the seven conditions and set of symptoms in the next section.

2. When you have done that, show your self-diagnosis to someone you trust. Then let her or him 'diagnose' you.
3. Compare the results.
4. Devise a treatment plan, or use the recommended ones at the end of the chapter.

While you are doing this exercise, remember that every leader has weaknesses and blind-spots. The key to preventing catastrophe is how the leader responds to these deficits, and how she or he treats the causes of the problem.

THE SEVEN CONDITIONS FOR LEADER FAILURE
Condition 1 – Blind-spots

A key characteristic of effective leaders is self-belief. But the stronger the belief, the more likely is it that leaders will be reluctant to give it up. For example, leaders may believe that they are capable of managing every aspect of a project. This belief persists, regardless of evidence to the contrary. The project fails, or runs out of steam. Leaders may blame others for the failure, and fail to understand their own role in events. In the worst cases leaders become dictators, in the process destroying their credibility and that of their followers. People who meet these leaders for the first time are confused by their seeming lack of grasp of reality. Let me give you an example.

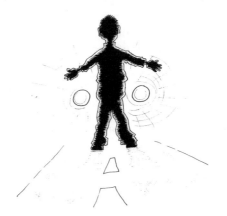

I don't see it … where?

Several years ago, I attended a meeting hosted by an adviser to an outgoing US President. The group I was with were staying at a hotel in central

Washington DC. Our meeting was at the White House. On our walk from our hotel to the meeting, we passed several homeless people. Some of the group had spoken to some of these homeless people on a previous occasion, to get another view of the American Dream. During our meeting, someone asked about the impact of the out-going Administration's economic policies. The homeless people we had seen and talked to were given as an example of people who had lost out in terms of jobs, wealth and homes. The reply we received was: 'You are wrong. There are no homeless people in Washington DC. People have never had it so good as under this Administration'.

After several seconds of chilling and stunned silence, we all began to protest (in that nice, British way which aims not to cause offence). Through this muted uproar, I watched the adviser. He honestly believed what he had said. In his eyes, *our* reality was faulty. Whatever the people living on the streets in the nation's capital city represented, they were not losers in an economic free-for-all. Other advisers we talked to, with one exception, all said more or less the same thing – 'We've done well, so why have people voted us out of office – the ingrates!' It was pure surrealism.

Personally, the most distressing thing about meeting people with such obvious blind-spots is the vertiginous sensation that I am losing what sense I have. When your view of reality is dismissed with implacable certainty, it takes time to regain a balanced view and re-focus on what you know to be fact, not just opinion. (I get the same sensation when I am told that racialism is not a problem in the NHS – it is just an idea put about by 'troublemakers' stirring up frenzy). Leaders with blind-spots create similar sensations in their followers. One end result is a deadening of sensitivity to those issues the leader cannot see or refuses to contemplate. After all, blind-spots protect us from having to re-order beliefs, or doubt ourselves. We are OK. It is other people who are out of step.

Symptoms

- Blames others for own failures.
- Believes that others are always wrong, stupid, or otherwise not as smart as she or he is.
- May seek scapegoats, or 'make examples' of others if things go wrong.
- Makes the same mistakes, in the same way, over and over and over again.
- Lacks self-awareness.
- Denies other people's reality.

Condition 2 – Just say yes

A leader undoubtedly has power over followers. Followers like to please the leader by doing what the leader wants. The closer the relationship between leader and follower, the greater the urge to please. This symbiotic relationship can lead to the creation of 'yes' men and women, which happens with alarming ease.

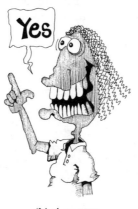

'Yes' woman

Put a group of people in a room together and the tendency is for them to try and agree with what each other is saying – if there are no deep divisions and hostilities within the group. This urge to please is magnified if followers believe that the leader can markedly affect their future in, for example, staff appraisal interviews. Paradoxically, over time unreflective 'yes' men and women become less valuable as sources of information. It is as if the leader has gained all the 'yes' required, and searches for a new supply.

In any event, both the leader and the yes-sayer mis-serve the other. The leader becomes divorced from reality, the yes-sayer becomes superfluous. Yes-saying can work both ways, with the leader screening out news that they believe will unsettle followers.

Symptoms

- Does not like people who disagree.
- Believes that disagreement is a sign of disloyalty.
- May tell 'little white lies' to try to protect followers from perceived harm.
- Apt to want to please those in positions of power.
- Believes that disagreements always cause conflicts.
- Apt to marginalize (or bully) dissenting followers, and perceive them as trouble-makers ('not a team player').

Condition 3 – Visions

Every leader needs a map or vision of where they want to go. Effective leaders share this map with their volunteers, and accept that modifications may be necessary. But when the leader's vision becomes indistinguishable from the leader's personal needs, they sometimes fail to see opportunities for developing their vision, or obstacles that will inhibit it.

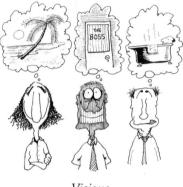

Visions

Conger relates the story of Edwin Land, inventor of the Polaroid camera (Conger 1990). Land's dream was to develop an automatic pocket-sized camera, one that would revolutionize instant photography. To achieve this, his personal vision, Land had to change the way his company conducted its business. For example, instead of contracting out the manufacture of this new camera, Land had to build a new factory and expand other facilities.

After several years, the new camera, the SX-70, was produced, and priced at $180.00. Expectation of sales in the first year, 1973, was several millions. But by the end of that year, only 470 000 cameras had been sold. Buyers just did not like the camera. Eventually, it sold in significant numbers, but only after several modifications which dispensed with many of the original features, and after a number of significant price-cuts.

Land's mistake was to believe that because people wanted instant photographs, they would buy his camera at any price. Why? Because *he* felt that way. An engineer at heart, he loved the technology of the product more than the actual product (what the customer bought) itself. In other words, Land became his camera, his vision.

Becoming their visions, such leaders ignore or do not listen to any view that is contrary to what they believe. Such behaviour can kill, as was shown by the destruction of the spacecraft, Challenger. Hearings into the incident suggested that some senior staff ignored warnings that there was a potentially fatal fault in the craft's fuel system. Sometimes the show must not go on.

Symptoms

- Apt to perceive the vision as their life's work, or personal legacy.
- Does not listen to contrary views of the vision.
- Has an exaggerated sense of the importance of the vision (for example, 'this new restructuring will solve all our problems').
- If the vision fails, is surprised and personally traumatized.

Condition 4 – Command and control

In an episode of *Star Trek: The Next Generation*, Picard, Dr Crusher and Worf are sent on a very secret mission by Starfleet. For the time they are away, the *Enterprise* is commanded by Captain Jellico. The remainder of the crew get ready to negotiate a treaty with the Cardassians. But they have a hard time understanding what Jellico expects of them. He accepts this, but insists that he has no time to explain anything. People must do as they are told.

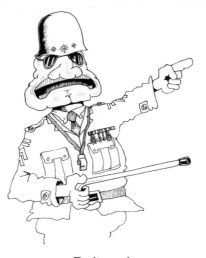

Do it now!

Before long, mutterings can be heard from the bridge to Ten Forward (the bar) by way of the cargo bays. Jellico is unmoved. Even Counsellor Troi has no luck – he listens to what she has to say, then tells her to dress more formally. The upshot of all this is that the Cardassians come dangerously close to calling off the negotiations, and almost succeed in scuppering the secret mission.

In an emergency, it is logical that people are ordered to act and be expected to obey. But leaders whose *normal* approach is command and control will not get the best from people. Remember situational leadership? The leader must adjust and adapt her or his style to the task in hand, to the maturity of followers, and to the desired outcomes of the project.

Symptoms

- Does not delegate.
- Is involved in the minutiae of the project.
- Apt to resent being asked to state explicit outcomes expected.
- Gives orders and expects obedience.
- Not very keen on followers taking initiative.
- Meddles in the work of followers.
- Eventually, burns out.

Condition 5 – Forgetting to lead

The first job of a leader is to lead. This includes appropriate delegation, not abdication. Remember the styles of leadership spectrum in Chapter 3? Too many leaders mistake delegation (entrusting a task or authority to another person) with abdication (renouncing responsibility).

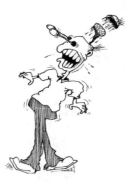

What, I'm the leader?!

Abdication is diametrically opposite to command and control. Each has value according to the job in hand. If the tool is not fit for, or is not adapted to, the purpose, then it is unlikely that the resulting product will be of sufficient quality to merit the time and energy spent on it. This is a basic tenet of any task fulfilment. Leaders frequently make assumptions about the capability of followers, without testing these assumptions. When followers do not meet the expected standard, the leader expresses disappointment, and may blame followers for their lack of application, or for apathy. I have heard many managers complain that their staff are lazy, apathetic, and only come to work for the money. Few have accepted that they are partly at fault, either through neglect of key factors such as acknowledging followers, or by not supplying the needed guidance or resources.

Forgetting to lead eventually damages the relationship between the leader and follower. Followers feel stranded, abandoned, and resentful. The leader may denigrate followers in private, and publicly. Neither side seems able to find mutual ground on which to rebuild. Examples of this cycle are prevalent in the NHS, and some of the symptoms can be seen easily:

Symptoms

- Lack of courtesy between leader and follower.
- In-fighting among followers.
- Loss of camaraderie; unhappiness.
- Unexplained increase in staff turn-over.
- Griping about the leader.
- Work-to-rule (that is, clock watching).
- Few, and irregular opportunities for followers' development.
- Little or no feedback on performance.

Condition 6 – Hubris

Hubris is a Greek word meaning arrogant pride or presumption. In Greek tragedy, hubris results in nemesis (or comeuppance). It is a near-fatal condition which affects leaders in the last stages of megalomania. Hubris was prevalent during the first years of the 1990 NHS reforms, a time which resembled a Greek tragedy (vainglorious talk, rank stupidity, and excessive pride). The comeuppance is now being received.

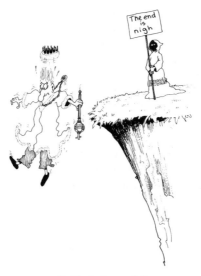

Pride before a fall

It is painful to watch a leader succumb to this condition. Many of the financial scandals in the NHS over the past few years have their basis in hubris, but blame is often apportioned to the workings of the internal market, as if the actors in those events had no mind, will, or ethics of their own. Hubris is one end result of a self-belief so strong that it defies rationality.

But healthcare leaders aren't the only ones susceptible to this terrible affliction. Pick up any newspaper and turn to the sports page and hubris is all over it – especially with regard to cricket, football, and lawn tennis. Perfectly sensible people, 'leading authorities in their field', talk the most arrant nonsense (the recent World Cup was one particularly notable example). Leaders who fall for hubris end up looking very silly. Pander to hubris, or lead. You cannot do both.

Symptoms

- Megalomania.
- Apt to use the jargon of the moment.
- Talks more than acts.
- Susceptible to flattery by 'experts'.
- Style of conversation not dissimilar to snake-oil salesman.
- Poor judgment.
- Believes that management consultants have the answer to every organizational ailment.

Condition 7 – Not saying goodbye

Sometimes leaders enjoy their work so much they cannot bear to think of anyone taking over their role. Yet as Conger argues, by centralizing power and authority around themselves, such leaders weaken an organization's authority structures (Conger 1990). No successors are reared, so the leader's vision dies on their departure.

Such leaders might have begun to perform below standard, but they so enjoy being the centre of attention that they cannot bear to leave the stage. The audience is dazzled more by their appearance than by their substance. They attend every conference, every meeting, whether it is appropriate or not. Followers get to do the boring stuff that the leader dislikes (such as attending low-profile community meetings). Followers may become dependent, and reluctant to take leadership roles.

Symptoms

- Hogs the limelight.

- Lack of attention to administration or detail.
- Highly dependent group of followers.
- Full diary of meetings outside the organization.
- Frequent absences for conferences.
- No development process for succession.

SUMMARY OF CONDITIONS AND SUGGESTED TREATMENT

Blind-spots. First identify them with the help of someone you trust. Then ask that person to deliberately challenge the blind-spots as they occur.

Yes-saying. Practise disagreeing with a person you usually agree with out of form. Note how you feel. Also ask people to disagree with you on specific issues. Note how you feel.

Visions. Give your vision away.

Command and control. This is a longterm treatment plan, requiring practice. Start by setting clear objectives for those you lead. Next, give them clear targets, with a date for feedback. But do not tell them how to do the tasks. Practise this until you are able to delegate the tasks with some authority.

Forgetting to lead. Ask those you lead what you are forgetting to do. Also, re-read Chapter 5 in this book.

Hubris. Stop before you start. If you have started, you might be beyond hope (this condition has a rapid progress). Find someone who is willing to hubris-watch, and alert you to signs of the condition.

Not saying goodbye. Repeat the treatment for Visions.

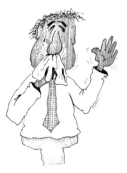

(Not) being able to say goodbye

Key learning points

- Every leader has weaknesses. It is how you deal with them that matters.

- The conspiracy against leadership is not inevitable.

- Leadership failure may be too high a price to pay for organizational dynamism.

- Learning from failure is a leadership characteristic.

REFERENCES

Argyris C 1991 Teaching smart people how to learn. Harvard Business Review 69(3): 99–109
Bennis W 1989 Why leaders can't lead: the unconscious conspiracy continues. Jossey-Bass, San Francisco
Caulkin S 1998 An audience with Warren Bennis, May: 76–77
Conger J 1990 The dark side of leadership. Organizational Dynamics 19(2): 44–55
Davidson L 1998 Alarm unheard or unheeded? Health Service Journal, June: 14–15
Kolb D A 1974 The process of experimential learning. In: Thorpe M, Edwards R, Hanson A (eds) Culture and processes of adult learning. p. 147
Limb M 1998 Board games. Health Service Journal, 10 July: 9

9

Leaders as transformers

Key words:

transformational leadership; gender; transactional leadership; continuous learning; self-development; managers and leaders

Looking on the bright side, failures in leadership can be minimized. Leaders will continue to have setbacks, but if these are used as opportunities to learn, then it is less likely that the same mistakes will be made again in the same way.

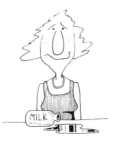

Look on the bright side

This is how leaders who are called 'transformational' approach their vision. They take a similar approach to people – what J. Sterling Livingston calls 'Pygmalion management' (Livingston 1988). Pygmalion was a sculptor from Greek mythology who carved a statue of a beautiful woman, who later came to life. In other words, he transformed her. George Bernard

Shaw turned Pygmalion into a play, and Hollywood turned it into the movie – *My Fair Lady*.

Remember the scene where Eliza Doolittle explains why Colonel Pickering is different from Professor Higgins? She says (Livingstone 1988):

The difference between a lady and a flower girl is not how she behaves but how she is treated. I shall always be a flower girl to Professor Higgins because he treats me like a flower girl. But I know I can be a lady to you because you always treat me like a lady and you always will.

Colonel Pickering types will always treat their volunteers in ways that improve their performance. The less said about the Professor Higgins type, the better – unintentionally or not, their behaviour towards staff leads to poor performance or under-achievement. Livingstone argues that both apathy and enthusiasm are infectious. Managers get what they give, and what they expect.

The study of transformational leadership dates from the early 1980s, and was partly driven by the resurgent women's movement of the 1970s, and partly by the increasing perception that business leadership was failing just at the time when companies threatened by recession needed leadership most.

In this chapter, we will look primarily at the making and development of transformational leaders, and whether anybody can become one. There is a short self-evaluation quiz at the end of the chapter, but I suggest you read Chapter 10 as well before you attempt it.

First, I want to set the context within research on leadership.

LEADERSHIP RESEARCH – A BRIEF HISTORY

Most of the research on leadership has been conducted in the USA, and has mainly focused on large companies in the private sector. Prior to 1973, the history of leadership was men studying men (that is, male researcher studying male managers). Models of leadership were based on the armed forces, leading to the construct of management and leadership (used interchangeably during this period) as command and control, the ascendancy of discipline and hierarchy, and the norm of managers as men. Companies like IBM spent millions of dollars training men for leadership of a type that was based on the leader as hero.

After 1973, leadership research began to consider women as managers and leaders in comparison to men. A resurgent feminist movement in the USA was a key driver of this research. But the researchers were still predominantly men, and the emphasis was still on men as the norm against which women were measured as managers and leaders.

A sea change occurred during the 1980s. More of the research on leadership was being conducted by women, and was providing women's perspective on leadership. Research studies now explicitly distinguished between leadership and management, and developed the concept of transformational leadership styles. The focus of this research was the different leadership styles of men compared with women, the first time that women had been the benchmarks for leadership.

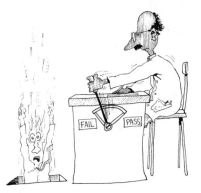

A failed leader or macho leadership?

A significant moment in research on transformational leadership came when the November/December 1990 issue of the *Harvard Business Review* carried an article called *Ways Women Lead*. The writer, Judy Rosener, presented the results of a survey sponsored by the International Women's Forum to investigate men and women leaders (we looked at Rosener's study earlier, in Chapter 3, but it bears a second visit). The survey uncovered differences in how women and men described their leadership performance, and therefore in how they lead:

 The men were more likely than the women to describe themselves in ways that characterize ... 'transactional' leadership [job performance as a series of transactions with subordinates] ... The women respondents, on the other hand, described themselves in ways that characterize 'transformational' leadership – getting subordinates to transform their own self-interest into the interest of the group through concern for a broader goal. (Rosener 1990)

To achieve their goals men tended to use rewards for good work and punishment for inadequate performance. Their power came from organizational position and formal authority. Conversely, women ascribed their sources of power to personal characteristics – charisma, hard work, interpersonal skills, or personal contacts. They relied less on organizational stature.

Rosener's article caused alarm to researchers who had never found such differences. Some doubted the accuracy of these descriptions which were, after all, self-reports. What did their followers have to say? Cue Professor

Bernard Bass, the leadership researcher's researcher, who surveyed 582 male and 219 female followers of 150 male and 79 female managers in six Fortune 500 companies. The results confirmed Rosener's findings:

> Women managers, on average, were judged more effective and satisfying to work for as well as more likely to generate *extra effort* [author's italics] from their people. Women were also rated higher than men on three of the 'Four Is' comprising transformational leadership. (Bass & Avolio 1994)

A common sense way to explain these differences is to conclude that women are more nurturing than men. Because they have been denied access to achieving organizational stature, they use their natural skills to the full. It just happens that these are the very skills that all organizations say they need to survive and thrive. The focus in now on putting such common sense views to the test, and expanding our understanding of the factors that comprise transformational leadership. As we have already discussed, UK researchers of leadership have begun to investigate transformational leadership as perceived in the National Health Service (NHS) and local government.

As research on transformational leadership increases, it is becoming clearer that to be transformational is to be female, or display the traits normally associated with (and sometimes denigrated in) women. But given that many of the women who broke through the 'glass ceiling' in organizations were obliged to play men's games to do it, there is probably a transformational deficit in many organizations.

One of the most significant phenomena of recent years is the number of small businesses started by women. In the USA, where this is most evident, more than 50% of all new jobs in the last decade have been in small business run by women. Many of these women were previously employed in large corporations. They quit because of boredom, lack of promotion, to have more time for themselves and their families, or to 'have an adventure' (Sherman 1994). Women appear to succeed better with such changes because our work patterns are curvy, compared with men's which, traditionally, have been linear. Women's work patterns mean that we are more adept at changing direction. We also accept our vulnerability and are used to expressing ourselves through feelings. These traits are common in transformational leaders. But what are these transformational leaders made of, and how do they get that way?

Let us recap on the identifying factors, the 'Four Is' of transformational leadership (Bass & Avolio 1994):

- Inspirational motivation – the leader uses symbols and simple emotional appeals to increase awareness of the vision.
- Idealized influence (charisma) – volunteers identify with and model themselves on their leader, whom they respect and trust.

- Individualized consideration – volunteers are treated differently but equitably on an individual basis.
- Intellectual stimulation – volunteers are encouraged, and supported, to challenge what they do and how they do it.

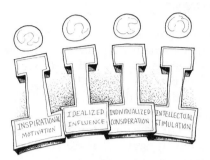

The Four Is

So, what do you do to become a transformational leader, and stay that way? As with most concepts, it is sometimes easier to describe it by what it is not.

TRANSFORMATIONAL AND DIFFERENT

From my observation, transformational leaders do not:

- Appear to be fond of those 'bonding' activities so popular in many organizations, and which are meant to improve team spirit (and which are just as likely to produce backbiting as to improve team work). So you would probably not find them walking over hot coals to prove anything, especially when they have seen others go before them and collapse in agony. Generally, leaders do not act against their best instincts.
- Make a show of their leadership – not their style.
- Steal their volunteers' glory, and hog the limelight.
- Stick rigidly to structures, procedures, or decisions which do not help them to achieve the vision.
- Believe in punishing volunteers for under-performance.
- Control others.
- Play favourites or exclude people from the vision.
- Place much emphasis on their status as a leader or anything else.
- Use information as a tactic to prevent other people from participating in the visions.
- Play psychological, or guessing, games.

We can reprise this list later, and some of these factors will be expanded when we talk about the Cardinal Sins of Leadership (Chapter 10). But having some idea of what transformational leaders are not, what is left? The 'Four Is' are a good place to start.

THE TRANSFORMERS

One result of the growing research on transformational leadership has been the design of instruments (mainly questionnaires) aimed at clarifying how the four factors of transformational leadership work in practice, looking especially at differences between men and women.

Bass and Avolio conducted three such studies using the Multifactor Leadership Questionnaire (MLQ), to examine followers' perceptions of male–female differences in transformational, transactional. and *laissez-faire* (that is, passive) leadership styles (Bass & Avolio 1996). Alimo-Metcalfe used an existing instrument, the Repertory Grid Technique, to conduct a study to identify what NHS and local government managers regard as transformational behaviours (we discussed this study in Chapter 3) (Alimo-Metcalfe 1996).

The main conclusions from such studies reinforced and expanded Rosener's ground-breaking work. In the Bass and Avolio studies, for instance, followers rated women leaders as exhibiting more transformational leadership behaviour than men. More significantly, women were just as likely as men to use transactional leadership styles (Bass and Avolio 1994). This was an important finding, because one of the reasons still given for women not acquiring senior management positions is our presumed inability to be tough, and manage poorly performing staff.

In *The Leadership Challenge*, Kouzes and Posner set out to discover how leaders actually practised leadership (Kouzes & Posner 1987, 1995). Their database took over 11 years to compile and contains information from 10 000 leaders and 50 000 followers. Kouzes and Posner identified five fundamental behaviours that successful leaders displayed. Not surprisingly, these five factors mirror the 'Four Is'. We will talk in more detail about Kouzes and Posner's research in Chapter 10. In the meantime, a summary of the five behaviours is presented in Box 9.1.

Box 9.1   The five practices of successful leaders (Kouzes & Posner 1995)

1. Inspiring a Shared Vision
2. Challenging the Process
3. Modelling the Way
4. Enabling Others to Act
5. Encouraging the Heart

Other general pieces of research on leadership also pinpoint key characteristics which mark transformational leadership behaviour. For example, in *The Fifth Discipline*, Peter Senge describes the new work, the new roles, and the new skills leaders need, to build learning organizations (a place where people are continuously learning). He also identifies some of the new tools necessary to achieve this goal (Senge 1990). According to Senge, the leader's new work is about creating opportunities for continuous learning. This starts with the principle of 'creative tension' – seeing where you are now ('current reality') and where you want to be ('the vision'). The gap between these two creates a natural tension.

Dr Martin Luther King Jnr, a great leader, employed this principle when he said that Americans must create 'the kind of tension in society that will help men rise from the dark depths of prejudice and racism'. Evidence-based healthcare practice also evokes the principle of creative tension.

The new roles of leaders are threefold:

- *Designer* – the behind-the-scenes activities that, though invisible, are vital to the success of any venture. For example, a poorly designed hospital will defeat the skills of the best practitioners. Organizational design starts with principles, values, and purpose, not structures, boxes, and lines.
- *Steward* – that is, the leader as the servant of followers. Remember the story of Mary Seacole in Chapter 2? Her whole life was one of wanting to serve others. Leaders who understand and take stewardship seriously ensure that their volunteers have the resources they need to accomplish the job. They are also stewards for the vision, the larger purpose that drives the job. If you are a fan of American football, consider this role as the one which protects the half-back (what I sometimes call 'running interference', or preventing obstruction), and enables him to pass the ball. In the case of leadership, the followers are the half-backs.
- *Teacher* – helping everyone involved, including yourself, to develop more insight and self-awareness.

To accomplish the new work and the new roles, leaders need new skills:

- Building a shared vision
- Testing mental models
- Systems thinking.

Taken together, much of the research on leadership is targeted at understanding how leaders and the organizations they work in can learn and grow together. This means an increasing emphasis on how leaders interact with, and impact, the groups they lead. We seem to be circling back to the human relations school of organization theory – people work best when they have some control over their work and are enabled to perform at high levels. The return to a kind of 'basics of leadership' is not surprising since the terms 'transactional and transformational leadership' were first used by James McGregor Burns more than 20 years ago. To quote:

... [when we] raise one another to higher levels of motivation and morality [transformational leadership occurs]. Their purposes, which might have started out as separate but related, as in the case of transactional leadership, become fused ... [But] transforming leadership ultimately becomes moral in that it raises the level of human conduct and ethical aspiration of both the leader and the led, and thus it has a transforming effect on both. (Senge 1990)

Clearly, Burns had a vision of what a transformational leader could accomplish. Two decades later, research has confirmed that this concept is not only valid, but is vital to achieving organizational and communal success.

What will we do with it? What do you need to do now to increase your ability to be a transformational leader, without losing your skills as a transactional leader? Like everything about leadership, you have to choose to make the transition.

CHOOSING TRANSFORMATION

Transformation does not choose you; you choose it. There are perfectly effective transactional leaders who treat their staff equitably, involve them in decision-making and generally run a 'good ship'. But the fault lines begin to show when obstacles occur, and a more flexible way of working is required.

Usually, obstacles present as changes of varying magnitude. The transactional leader, used to accomplishing objectives through wielding power and position, finds it difficult to let staff be in charge of the change that affects them. The transformational leader, accustomed to sharing power, using influence, and developing potential, has probably spotted the change before it happened. Both leaders will survive, but only the transformational leader is likely to have implemented a lasting change.

The leadership challenge facing nurse leaders is the transformation of health care on three levels – for patients, for the development of nursing, and for self-development.

Challenge 1 – Transforming health care for patients

When the Patient's Charter was first published, I remember feeling quite insulted and angry that a group of primarily non-nurses were telling me how to treat *my* patients. Of course my anger was really directed at myself and my colleagues, who had too often failed to treat patients with respect, courtesy and dignity. Since then we have come to know just how badly some patients are treated – racialism, lack of knowledge about non-Christian religious needs and rituals, and a general failure to humanize health care.

If patients are to have positive experiences in their contact with health services, then nurse leaders must develop services which have the patient at the centre of the process. Some of the big things which will help include:

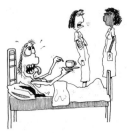

Please, please, all I want is a cup of tea!

- A *quality of service* which is based on what each patient says is a quality service. Complex models of care will never take the place of listening to what patients tell us about their view of their illness, or need for care.
- An *ethical base* to all care given is axiomatic. Yet in fields such as mental health, midwifery and learning disabilities, the ingrained paternalism in nursing leads to distress and sometimes harm to patients. For example, forcing a woman to have a Caesarean section is not only unethical, but a breach of our obligation to do our patients no harm.
- *Research* which takes account of patients' experiences. The continuing emphasis on biomedical research leaves little room for alternate methods – personal stories, biographies, folk tales, allegory. One of the most striking outcomes of the RCN Ward Leadership programme is that participants re-discovered the importance of sitting and talking to patients. Research must always move us closer to our patients, not further away from them.
- *Patient teaching*. The expert on any condition is the person who has it. The very least we can do is seek their help to get the facts right. Some spe-cialist areas have done this for years, especially in gynaecology – women who have experienced a certain condition share these experiences with oth-ers in a similar state. But there is another area of patient teaching which is under-developed – that of patients teaching the professionals. There is at least one pioneering scheme in the UK (based in Cambridge), several in the USA, and a few across Scandinavia. The participants being taught are usu-ally medical students (who apparently have a greater need for this type of activity than nurses). The initial response is usually reluctance, quickly fol-lowed by a natural willingness to relieve ignorance. Such schemes for mid-wifery and nurse students are overdue.
- *Patient involvement* in as many aspects of service monitoring, audit and review as possible. This is dependent on level of interest, but have you noticed how the patient does not seem to have more than a peripheral role in the clinical governance, clinical effectiveness, and service audit initia-

tives? It serves little purpose to bombard patients with questionnaires about (usually) their stay in hospital. Not only do they never hear about the results, they are rarely involved in designing the questionnaire. Many hospitals and GP practices have patient groups, and no doubt, the community health councils play their part. The reality is that most patients do not care a pinch about their care – they trust us not to harm them. But if we want to get all sides of the story, we need to ask patients how they want to be involved. For example, in one ante-natal clinic, women expressed a wish to complete, for themselves, the front cover of the notes. One result of adopting this idea was a marked decrease in the misspelling of names and addresses and the incorrect recording of telephone numbers. More generally, many patients now carry their medical records, with a corresponding decrease in lost notes and the recording of denigrating remarks.

● *Community education and development.* By this, I mean enabling local people to take better care of their health and their environment. Beyond health education and health promotion, community education and development falls in the category of social entrepreneurship. We know that a community's health is a function of education, economics and other social processes. Community nursing is well developed in the UK, but educating communities is not. The new primary care groups (PCGs) may be a key to developing this concept (that is, if PCGs don't degenerate into a more malevolent form of fundholding). But this can only happen if whoever represents nurses, midwives and health visitors on the PCG board is willing to consider that definitions of 'primary care' do not begin and end with a general practitioner.

● *'Team work'* is the word of this passing century. Most job descriptions demand it, and most of us think it is a good idea. With apologies to Groucho Marx, any club which has such a need of new members is one I am not particularly keen to join. Team work takes a long time to develop, the prime requirement being exemplary leadership. But if we are to improve the healthcare experience for patients, we have to talk to each other, work together, and give up territory. We also have to respect each other's differences (from skin colour to political views), and rapidly learn the art of disagreeing with a view without disliking the person. I am not saying that we must love all our colleagues, but there is a wider interest than our egos at stake. We say we are 'here for the patient' – but our actions must always speak louder than our words.

After the big things, some of the little things which, when present, can help make daily frustrations more bearable:

● Little common courtesies (for example, 'please', 'thank you', 'excuse me', 'may I help you?', 'I will find someone who can help you')
● Nutritious food
● Premises in good repair
● Sheets and pillows

- Equipment that works (telephones, lights, lifts, ice machines)
- Readable and accessible signposting, in various languages
- Staff wearing name badges (including consultants)
- Bed linen
- Letters which carry the signature of the writer
- Enough coffee, tea and sugar to last for more than one shift
- Waste paper bins emptied at least daily.

Make up your own list. Patients are probably the first to notice when the little things start being missed in the daily routine. Having twice been a patient, the boredom of ward life is relieved by watching how the staff work with each other. You also have time to stare at peeling ceilings, follow the tracks of bed fluff, count the number of missing hooks on the curtain rails around the bed, and guess who is on duty by the number of times the phone rings before being answered. If we want to transform patient care, maybe we should start by asking the recipient.

Challenge 2 – Transforming nursing

Every decade or so, someone has a 'new idea' that aims to reduce the numbers of people leaving nursing. The latest is the nurse consultant. While the idea of nurse consultants is neither new nor controversial, it alone cannot bear the load of spearheading the radical transformation that is required if health visitors, midwives and nurses are to be part of the kaleidoscope of partnerships that will influence the shape of health and social care in the next millennium.

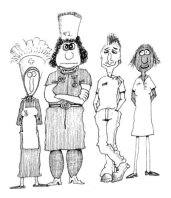

Transformation

Neither will Project 2000 provide much of an answer. Pre-registration preparation of all healthcare workers will have to move closer to our business – patients, especially those with increasingly specialized needs.

At least one set of educators have positioned themselves for this future: Queen Mary and Westfield College, in conjunction with Tower Hamlets Healthcare Trust in London recently advertised for a Project Coordinator for a community based teaching programme, initially targeted at medical students (*The Guardian*, 23 September 1998). A novelty? No, because it has long been unviable to pack student nurses, doctors or other healthcare workers into separate classrooms, in separate parts of a hospital or university, only letting them loose on each other, and on patients, after 4 to 7 years of varying degrees of indoctrination. Not viable, and guaranteed to perpetuate stereotypes, lack of understanding of roles, and general hostility of one to the other.

To transform nursing means transforming nurse education. One possible future scenario is to have no entrants to pre-registration nursing programmes who are younger than 21 years old. The older the better. Demographics are already running against us in this regard. Instead of worrying about the drop in the number of teenagers wanting to enter nursing, we should plan to optimize the skills and motivation of the nurses we already have. We should also expect that recruits have a wide education base, work experience, and wider interests beyond health care. In other words, we want renaissance nurses. And when we get them, we have to work to keep them.

But what has been the response to the continuing exodus of nurses from the NHS – recruit from overseas. I have no doubt that there are skill shortages in many areas of nursing, but the sticking plaster that is overseas recruiting is no answer. By and large, nursing remains hierarchial, introverted, defensive, and fearful of change. Where are the innovative ideas to get and keep midwives, nurses, and health visitors? Do we know why such people leave their profession in such increasing numbers every year? Money must be one issue, but not the only one. Some others might include:

- Poor management
- Top-down management
- Racialism
- Inflexible shift patterns
- Poor development and promotion opportunities
- Increased stress due to lack of control over work
- Better things to do
- Inflexible approach to work-breaks
- Boredom
- Lack of leadership
- Lack of support for innovation
- Inadequate attention to recruitment and retention.

The midwives, nurses and health visitors who do stay learn how to 'cope', but those who strive for innovative practice may find themselves accused of rocking the boat.

After nearly 2 decades of experimentation with markets, the NHS has 'rediscovered' patients and with them midwives, nurses and health visitors. This might be to our benefit, if we know what to do with the attention. Generally, nurses have had little influence on policy. White has argued that nurses do not know how to use power:

> ... nurses have had little manifest power in the past, have not known how to use what little power they had, and so have learned to prefer an oblique approach rather than become embroiled in a frontal attack. We tend to go around, or surmount, difficulties rather than to confront them. We are better at reacting than proacting ... on the whole we are not very brave at confronting reality. [But] this is changing ... (White 1988)

We still get into difficulties when trying to define nursing (or midwifery, or health visiting). Everyone, it seems, has a definition of what a nurse is and does. For our part, we have often allowed others to dictate our role. But whatever we are, we are not a unitary occupation with one set of goals and a single value system. White found three sub-groups among nurses (White 1988):

1. The *managers*, who control nursing staff, provide nursing services within constrained budgets, and uphold the status quo from which they get their authority.
2. The *generalists*, who are in nursing to earn a living. They have much in common with managers as they are satisfied with the status quo and not overly concerned to increase professional authority or their knowledge base.
3. The *specialists*, who want to have professional authority based on higher education and specialized knowledge, and control the whole process of nursing. They tend to challenge the status quo and are therefore often in conflict with managers and generalists.

Such categories are not fixed, but peer group pressure in nursing is strong. Change-minded managers may find it difficult to maintain such a stance in the face of status-quo-minded colleagues. A graduate nurse may share values similar to the generalists. But policy-makers continue to regard nursing as unitary, and so have nursing organizations. Hence the focus on 'pay and rations' with, until recently, little attention being given to professional authority.

The plural society that characterizes nursing needs a plural approach to leadership. Why not have different entry routes for the different groups? The police and the civil service have accelerated development programmes for those who are its future leaders, and technical specialists. The NHS has its accelerated programme for management. Could the RCN's Ward Managers programme develop into something similar for nurses, et al?

But we need more than programmes. We need people with passion for their profession, a drive to innovate, and the optimism to see opportunity where others see obstacles. One of the areas where we need this energy is in research.

It is revealing that, while bio-medical research is well established and well funded, health services research (the kind that targets outcomes, organization behaviours, qualitative issues, and has little monetary value) comprises a very small percentage of research activity in the NHS, and among nurses. But without this kind of research, it will be almost impossible to create innovative practice in patient care.

We have very few qualitative research projects on nursing leadership. This is changing slowly, especially in relation to shared leadership or shared governance, which is based on (yet another) US management concept. A handful of sites are pioneering this concept, including St. George's Healthcare Trust in Tooting, Pontefract Hospitals NHS Trust, West Yorkshire. Other sites are in North Devon, Ipswich and Leicester.

Shared governance was first used in the US motorcar industry to give auto workers greater involvement in decision-making. The concept has been adapted to nursing by Tim Porter O'Grady, Canadian nurse entrepreneur (Naish 1995). The Tavistock Institute in London pioneered work in shared governance, but it's only in the last few years that UK organizations have taken any interest.

In a nutshell, shared governance aims to actively involve those at the frontline in the decisions about what they do, and how it is done. As a consequence, people will know the importance of their role in the whole enterprise, and will gain increased levels of accountability. The NHS sites which are using shared governance appear to focus on changing practice, but also use this as an opportunity to develop skills that will take nurses outside their usual boundaries (Leifer 1997, Legg & Hennessy 1996).

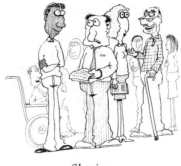

Sharing

Shared governance is probably one of the few radical ideas currently circulating in nursing, and could have a major impact on nursing practice. It presents nurses with another opportunity to refine the role, purpose and function of nursing. It challenges assumptions about who owns knowledge, who has power, and who has the right to make decisions. It therefore reflects transformational leadership, and has the potential to enhance the new entrepreneurial spirit which is evident in many areas of nursing.

Challenge 3 – Transforming self

In recent years, life-long learning has been urged on us by governments and by employers. Put simply, if we keep on learning, then we are more likely to succeed at what we do, and are more able to handle uncertainty and rapid change.

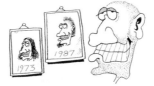

Transformation

Nurses have always valued development, usually in the form of courses and qualifications. The problem it that much of that development has been scatter gun, not sniper fire. For self-development to aid learning, it must have the intent to create a capacity for reflection, risk-taking and transforming self. There are many ways you can transform your learning and your life without attending any more courses, or getting any more qualifications, but our own natures can act against us. Try Exercise 9.1 to see what I mean:

Exercise 9.1

Find a quiet place. Relax. For 5 minutes try to concentrate on only one thought or idea. (Remember to make a note of the time you started and finished.)

It should be no surprise if you found that 5 minutes was not as short (or as long) as you thought. The whole focus of what we do in health care is motion – meetings, reporting, treatments, writing, transporting. In times past, nurse students were 'told off' for sitting and talking to patients. I understand that talking to patients is still frowned upon by the Taylorite tendency in nursing. But if we do not sit still, how will we hear ourselves?

Imagine sitting all day on a platform at a busy railway station like Clapham Junction – banging doors, whistles, the garbled tannoy system, people talking/shouting/screaming, pigeons doing their thing, trains entering, leaving and passing through the station. Multiply these sounds by any number and you would still not get close to the amount of noise that goes on in our heads every day.

The human brain is like a huge Clapham Junction. Everything we do is noted, calculated, and stored. So we need to ensure that what we put in is high quality, because whatever goes in comes out.

I recently read somewhere that on average, a manager receives more information in one day than was available to whole countries less than 30 years ago. Technology has increased the amount of available information; I am not sure it has improved the quality. We need regular periods of time-out, turning down the volume of all that activity for several minutes a day to boost energy levels and relieve stress. A few ideas on how to achieve this follow, starting with reflection.

REFLECTION

For several years, reflection has provided a framework for self-development and practice development processes in many professions. For nurses, reflection is part of the preparation for registration with the UKCC, and is being used in clinical supervision. Managers have also discovered that reflection can be a powerful source of energy and insight. Several organizations in the UK routinely use meditation as a development tool (but they do not publicize this, especially not to shareholders). Some US companies see reflection as a skill which can be acquired. It may be this decade's fad, but people who are comfortable with not striving for answers (that is, being introspective or reflective) are more likely to let you do the same. Reflection also enables us to learn from mistakes and move on.

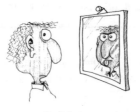

Reflection

Punishment, and demanding leaders, can only go so far in driving change. If individuals do not develop the capacity to reflect, they might not be able to respond quickly to change, and therefore ensure their survival. We do reflect on our actions, but to receive lasting benefit the reflection needs to be systematic. There are several books written on the subject, but a simple method is to keep a daily diary of events – as does *Star Trek*'s Captain's Log.

Reflection can take many forms – talking through an event with colleagues, meditation, yoga, several forms of martial arts, writing a daily diary, creating different scenarios for events that have happened or are about to happen (like getting ready for an interview), questioning your values and beliefs, staring into space. Learning to reflect requires a willingness to be objéctive, honest with yourself, and to focus on learning. In a *Fortune* magazine article, Stratford Sherman (1994) suggests that there are nine goals for successful introspection (which I see as intensive reflection). I have expanded on Sherman's goals and added another four (numbered 10–13). They are all outlined in Box 9.2.

Box 9.2   The 13 goals of successful introspection

1. *Objectivity* – reflection must be based on reliable information. Get data from as many people as possible. Explicitly ask colleagues and others to confront you about those areas about which you may have blind-spots, or in which you lack confidence.
2. *Responsibility* – take responsibility for your actions, and for your state of mind. To paraphrase the *I Ching*, an inferior person blames others for their misfortune and difficulties. But the superior person 'seeks the error within [her or himself], and through this introspection the external obstacle becomes ... an occasion for inner enrichment and education'.
3. *Action* – be able to respond to change, and act on your values.
4. *A balanced life* – family, friends, work, socializing are all important. But work life is increasingly stressful. Setting priories is never easy, but the attempt can prevent Pyrrhic victories. If you have difficulty remembering the last time you had a carefree day, check the balance in your life.
5. *Self-confidence* – not false courage, but a willingness to handle your emotions, no matter how painful, and know your strengths and vulnerabilities. This is not California dreaming, but a necessary part of self-development.
6. *Learning* – introspection must result in continuous learning. Senge talks about balancing inquiry (asking questions) and advocacy (supporting a particular position). Only by using both these skills can learning take place. (Senge 1990) (Learning is a process that produces a relatively permanent change in behaviour.)
7. *Tolerance for ambiguity and uncertainty* – you can never have all the facts before deciding to act. The future you hope will be better does not exist – you have to make it up as you go along. Success with this goal is the key to living with paradox.
8. *Creativity and intuition* – most education systems (based on logic, systems, analysis, hierarchy) are focused on the left brain. Many of us are therefore only functioning as half a person. Get the right side of your brain active, if only by watching *Star Trek*, and imagining how you would deal with that glowing life form who speaks in riddles.
9. *Egolessness* – try to act and take decisions without putting your needs first. Unfortunately, many nurses excel at this. Express your needs, concerns, desires openly, and then act. You will feel less guilty and frustrated.
10. *Laugh at yourself* – if you bore yourself, you will certainly bore others. Never take yourself seriously. But take what you do seriously.
11. *Crap detecting* – necessary when reading any article or book on self-development. Read to clarify your thoughts, not to reinforce your feelings of unworthiness before gurus.
12. *Pinch of salt* – take everything with a.
13. *Self-interest* – if you are not prepared to spend time and money on your own self-development, why should anyone else?

You can practise introspection anywhere, anytime. But to get the benefit, it must become a regular part of your life. Below are some other suggestions for taking breaks from your routines:

- Physical exercise – the sort that makes you sweat.
- Stare into space.
- Read a book about a subject, or by an author, you know nothing about.
- Cook the most exotic, or the simplest, meal you can. Both need creativity.
- Learn a new skill or language, or refresh a current one.
- Learn to meditate.
- Sing along to your favourite songs – out of tune. It will make you laugh.
- Do something frivolous.
- Lock yourself in the house and give yourself undivided attention.
- Go shopping – and buy nothing.
- Watch your children (or any children) playing, talking, or just being children.
- Go singing in the rain.
- Take a train or bus to anywhere.
- Depending on your habit, watch television indiscriminately or discriminately.
- Dance.
- Watch a talk show and be thankful.
- Watch the shopping channel.
- Cultivate anarchic thoughts.
- Say 'I love you' to the mirror.
- Sleep.

BECOMING A TRANSFORMATIONAL LEADER – THE QUIZ

The quiz is based on the dimensions of transformational leadership we first discussed in Chapter 3 (Bass and Avolio's 'Four Is', Kouzes and Posner's five fundamentals of exemplary leadership, Alimo-Metcalfe's research for the Local Government Management Board). The aim of the exercise is for you to reflect on your transformational leadership behaviour, and plan how to improve your transformational leadership behaviour.

There are 10 statements, each of which carries 10 points. For each response to each statement, mark yourself out of 10, depending on how well you believe you do each activity now (0 is 'not at all', 10 is 'totally and completely'). The score card at the end of Part I of the quiz is a guide to what you need to do to increase transformational leadership behaviour.

Quiz – Part 1

1. Transformational leaders are role models. They are respected and trusted by their volunteers, and set the standard for others to follow. How well do I do this now?

2. Exemplary leaders inspire people, give them a goal to aim for and support them while they are working towards it. How am I doing?

3. To keep morale high, transformational leaders celebrate successes, and give volunteers praise and recognition for their work. How much of this do I do, and how well?

4. Leaders challenge the status quo, and encourage experimentation and innovation. They are entrepreneurs who take calculated risks to achieve their vision. How am I doing?

5. Exemplary leaders form partnerships and make alliances, and use delegation as a way of developing their volunteers. They are more interested in sharing information than in protecting their territory. How well do I do this?

6. Actively supporting individuals' development is a mark of transformational leaders. This can happen in many ways, including encouraging independent thinking, challenging values and beliefs, and through assignments which focus on building knowledge and self-confidence. How am I doing?

7. Transformational leaders willingly admit their mistakes, viewing them as learning experiences. They are also self-aware and try to maintain a balance between their needs and those of their volunteers. How well am I performing on this?

8. Transformational leaders are creative thinkers who can see both the 'big picture' and the detail, and can grasp complex issues. How is my performance on this?

9. Exemplary leaders have strongly held core values which they do not compromise. Have I, and do I?

10. Transformational leaders use political skills to bring together the key players needed to achieve goals. They maintain effective working relationships with these groups and are sensitive to their interests and priorities. How am I doing?

Score card

20 and below: You may be underestimating yourself, or peer pressure prevents you from improving. If not, you may have unhappy staff or colleagues, and are finding your job difficult to do. If you want to change, start by explicitly asking three colleagues you trust (any more might get up your nose) to give you honest feedback about how you work. Use that information to change one thing at a time about yourself. This might take some time, but persevere. If you choose not to change – where did you say you worked?

21–40: You have known that you need to do more to change your behaviour as a leader. In becoming more transformational, you may find it useful to focus on the two or three behaviours which you find particularly difficult and ask for explicit feedback from a small group of trusted colleagues or friends. Also include time for reflection in your week.

41–60: You are exhibiting many transformational leadership behaviours. What you need to do now is actively develop these behaviours, giving particular attention to those which you may be doing unconsciously. You also need to make time for reflection on how you lead and how you want to develop further.

61–80: You clearly have well-established transformational leadership behaviours. Now, how do you keep them? It would be easy to think that you have almost 'made it'. You therefore need to be conscious that you are a transformational leader. Be aware of what your values are, how these are articulated, and what might compromise them.

81–100: Obviously and knowingly a transformational leader. Are you a mentor, coach, or teacher? If not, why not?

Quiz – Part 2

Ask five people you trust to score you on the questions in Part I of the quiz. Take an average for each dimension to get their total score. Compare their scores with yours. The greater the difference, the more conscious you need to be of how your behaviour as a leader is perceived by others.

Whatever your score, you need to work with a mentor and/or coach, someone who will challenge you to sustain your development as a leader. Transformational leadership is a mind set, but you have to set your mind to it.

Key learning points

- Transformational leadership is a mind set, rather than a competency.
- Research on transformational leadership suggests that women are more likely than men to describe themselves as having transformational behaviours.

Key learning points (*cont'd*)

- There are significant differences between US and UK findings on the dimensions on transformational leadership.

- Nurse leaders need to adopt transformational behaviours to transform patient care, nursing, and themselves.

- Reflection is a primary part of becoming a transformational leader.

- Every leader needs a mentor or a coach.

REFERENCES

Alimo-Metcalfe B 1996 Leaders or Managers? Nursing Management 3(1): 22–24
Bass B M, Avolio B J 1994 B J Shatter the glass ceiling: women may make better managers. Human Resource Management 33(4): 549–560
Bass B M, Avolio B J 1996 The transformational and transactional leadership of men and women. Applied Psychology: An International Review 45(1): 5–34
Kouzes J M, Posner B Z 1987 The leadership challenge: how to get extraordinary things done in organizations. Jossey-Bass, San Francisco
Kouzes J M, Posner B Z 1995 The leadership challenge: how to keep getting extraordinary things done in organizations. Jossey-Bass, San Francisco
Legg S, Hennesy M 1996 Fair shares in practice. Nursing Management 2: 6–7
Leifer D 1997 New way of leading. Nursing Standard 11(51): 12
Livingstone J S 1988 Pygmalion in management. Harvard Business Review 66(5): 121–130
Naish J Give up your power. Nursing Management 2(2): 7
Rosener J B Ways women lead. Harvard Business Review 68(6): 119–125
Senge P M 1990 The fifth discipline: the art and practice of the learning organization. Doubleday, New York
Sherman S 1994 Leaders learn to heed the voice within. Fortune 110(4): 64–70
White R 1988 Political issues in nursing: past, present and future, vol 3. John Wiley, Chichester

10

The 10 steps of leadership

Key words:

cardinal sins; sex, but no lies; the *Star Trek* code of leadership

SEX, LIES AND LEADERSHIP

Leaders face many temptations, not least of which are the ones of arrogance, overweening self-confidence, and succumbing to hubris. But probably the greatest temptation is that which accompanies the need to maintain the image of a leader.

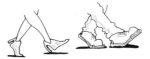

By now you know that your image of what a leader is or should be is self-created. It is built upon selected experience of leaders, prevailing notions of leadership, power and authority (accepted or rejected), and a smattering of wish fulfilment. How you decide to lead is a composite of these elements (and more), your set of values, your beliefs and your personality.

In this chapter, I want to focus on the work of James Kouzes and Barry Posner. Kouzes and Posner's work is of more than academic interest. The people they interviewed for their study were actual leaders doing the job of leading. If you already know about their research on leaders, then the text may give you an opportunity to think about their work in more depth. If their work is new to you, then welcome (and why haven't you read

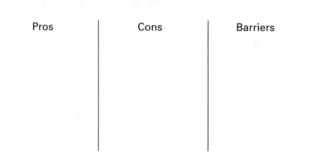

Figure 10.1 Fundamentals of exemplary leadership.

Chapter 3 and Chapter 9 yet?). In any event, I want us to consider how what Kouzes and Posner say about the 'five fundamental practices of exemplary leadership' can be applied to health and social care settings, whether clinical or managerial. I will then suggest that there are nine things (or behaviours) that leaders cannot indulge in, and still expect to portray exemplary leadership and keep and recruit volunteers.

Before we start, I would like you to do the following:

- Get a few sheets of A4 paper, enough to provide the headings for the five fundamentals of exemplary leadership.
- As we explore the fundamentals, make three columns for each heading, to represent Pros, Cons, and Barriers. An example of what I mean is set out in Figure 10.1.
- At the end of our exploration, make an honest assessment of the barriers you believe would prevent you from achieving each of the fundamentals. Write these in the Barriers column.

THE EXEMPLARY LEADER

According to Kouzes and Posner, there are five 'fundamental practices' which are necessary for exemplary leadership. By using the word exemplary (which they use interchangeably with 'extraordinary'), Kouzes and Posner are talking about leaders who are outstanding in their performance and attitude to leadership. In fact, the subtitle of their now famous book (*The Leadership Challenge*) is *How to Keep Getting Extraordinary Things Done in Organizations* (Kouzes & Posner 1995).

From their research, Kouzes and Posner have concluded that the following five practices define exemplary leadership:

1. Inspiring a shared vision
2. Enabling others to act
3. Challenging the process
4. Encouraging the heart
5. Modelling the way.

These five elements have been further split into the 10 Commitments of Leadership, which are simply behaviours that extraordinary leaders exhibit. They include building trust, practising what you preach, and ensuring that people are competent to do the job in hand. The full list of the fundamentals and the 10 Commitments is given at the end of this chapter.

As Table 10.1 shows, the five fundamentals that Kouzes and Posner developed, have parallels with Bass and Avolio's 'Four Is' of transformational leadership (Bass & Avolio 1994).

Table 10.1   Parallels between Kouzes and Posner's five fundamentals and Bass and Avolio's Four Is of transformational leadership

Five fundamentals of leadership	The Four Is of transformational exemplary leadership
1. Inspiring a shared vision	Inspirational motivation
2. Enabling others to act	Individualized consideration
3. Challenging the process	Intellectual stimulation
4. Encouraging the heart	Idealized influence (or charisma)
5. Modelling the way	No perfect match but equivalent to integrity, which is implicit in the Four Is

But how do the five fundamentals work in practice? In a busy ward, clinic or board room, how do you find the time to be an exemplary leader? Let's take each of the fundamentals and test them in situations which are common to health and social care. We need to do this not only because Kouzes and Posner focused primarily on leaders in the private sector, but also to see how ideas about leadership are translated across social cultures. Remember that, as with any other idea, leadership has a social as well as an organizational context.

1. Inspiring a shared vision

Kouzes and Posner give examples of visionary leaders that make me drool: the woman who led the first American climbing team to reach the summit of the 10th highest mountain in the world; the company that involved all 3400 employees in inventing a future for the company; the high school in Houston which uses a unique combination of self-discovery techniques and students' memories of their mothers to teach construction to a class of difficult students. These are examples of how inspirational leaders can encourage us to rise above our perceived limitations and be better than we believe we can be.

Who would argue that to accomplish anything, it helps if the participants are enthusiastic about what they are doing, and believe they are part of something bigger than themselves? Visionary leaders have the capacity to invent the future, and imagine a more ideal state than the present.

Put yourself in this position. You have a strong desire to do something challenging, whether in your personal life or at work. You eat, sleep, and breathe this idea to the point of obsession. Eventually you get a clearer idea for what the challenge is, and you begin to plan to achieve it. You gather information, put a cost on your idea, and maybe write down what you want to achieve. You sell your idea to a few people, emphasizing the benefit they will get from joining your project. Gradually your idea becomes reality, your determination to succeed grows, and so does your desire to change more things.

Every major change has had its start in somebody's vision of the future, and has gone through a process like the one I have just described – whether the vision is positive or negative, the process is the same. Visions of the future are about possibilities which, unlike probabilities, require no evidence that they will succeed. As such, visions are suggestions of how the future could be. They require no resources except your energy, sleepless nights, and the loss of acquaintances who get fed up with your quibbling about quality or some other obsession.

Without visionary leaders, we are unlikely to get the improvements we say we want to make our lives better – education, health care, civil life, street cleaning, breathable air, better movies, less crap television. Yet visionary leaders have not always had the praise they have enjoyed of late. One former US President (George Bush) spoke almost disparagingly about 'the vision thing'. Macho managers who believe that employees should do as they are told and not ask any questions about where the organization is going are not fond of the 'V' word. After all, who wants a pack of busybody, nit-picking and nosy workers mucking about with that nice strategy which only senior managers are entitled to see?

The trouble with visionary leaders is they always want things to be different. That might be OK in a country like the USA, where people seem to be forever changing their address and their identities. In a society which is generally uneasy with change, and more at ease with the status quo, visionary leaders may have to work harder to be inspirational.

In practice, inspiring a vision of the future depends as much on the leader as on the people willing to share the vision. Some leaders may strive for several years and never get their idea off the ground. If you ever find yourself in this position, stop digging a hole for yourself and re-focus your vision. Inspiring a vision also depends upon:

- *Your integrity in owning the vision.* If your vision is a fake, you will be found out.
- *The relevance of the vision to the lives of the people whose support you need.* Would you follow someone in whom you did not believe?
- *Timing.* Some visions are obvious to others only at times of crisis, for

example, when there is a nursing shortage and there is a scramble to find 'innovative ways' to increase retention of experienced nurses (and midwives).

- *How you sell your story.* It helps if you have real passion for your dream.
- *How you make up your vision as you go along.* A vision is simply a made-up future that you are aiming for. It is not real – embellish, embroider, and go for broke.
- *Your willingness to give your vision away.* The future you dream about will take more than you, and maybe more than one lifetime, to achieve.

Health care is in desperate need of visionary leaders, people who are passionate about, and committed to creating a better health service. They are there, saying the wrong things, asking awkward questions, running against the herd instinct prevalent in every organization. They dream about having mental health services which provide sanctuary and healing, as well as meeting public demands for safety. They talk at length (sometimes obsessively) of creating collaborative working partnerships, not because politicians say they should, but because that is the most effective way to use scarce resources and provide high quality services. They will laugh at the false starts they have had, and tell you about the plans they have for turning a derelict building into a breakfast and after-school club (in part-nership with local people). Working with such people can be exhausting, until you change jobs and discover how rare they are, and its only then that you learn to appreciate them

Everyone is inspired by something, and dreams of making a difference. What marks leaders is their commitment to go the distance with their visions, and for the people they enlist in the effort. Which brings me to the next fundamental: enabling others to act.

2. Enabling others to act

To quote Kouzes and Posner (1995):

In more than 550 original cases we studied, we didn't encounter a single example of extraordinary achievement that occurred without the active involvement and support of many people ... from all professions and from around the globe, people continue to tell us, 'You can't do it alone, It's a team effort'.

Exemplary leaders enable others to act by:

- Strengthening others through sharing power and information (being sensitive, developing everyone's competence, building others' self-esteem, increasing decision-making authority, providing visible support).

- Fostering collaboration through mutual trust and cooperative goals (emphasizing longterm payoffs, fostering reciprocity, seeking integrative solutions, improving performance, promoting and sustaining durable interactions – dealing with people on a longterm basis).

Does this remind you of anything? Remember Elton Mayo's argument that a manager's job is to engender spontaneous cooperation, thus reducing the basis for conflict between the 'logic of sentiment' and the 'logic of cost and efficiency'? Enabling others does not mean advocacy or being Mother Earth. To enable others, leaders build on a variety of behaviours and attitudes, like giving people control of their destiny, and showing respect for others' opinions and differences.

You cannot do it alone. You do not, and never will, have all the skills, knowledge, information, energy and networks to accomplish any task. Forget that nurses are still 'raised' to cope. Leaders do *not* cope. They enable others to help them achieve their goals. They do this by fostering mutual trust, building collaborative relationships, creating mutual goals, and developing give-and-take in interactions (that is, reciprocity). The last is especially important to health care, as the complexity of the issues we need to address requires a huge level of face-to-face communication. If you know that you will be having serial communication with a colleague, you are obliged to maintain a positive relationship with them. This way you are both better able to reconcile your differences, and build mutual confidence, cooperation, and respect.

An unwillingness to collaborate produces the sort of conflict which is evident between countries (Palestine and Israel), between races (practically every country), and within organizations (terminal deadlock over needed changes). When leaders meet situations like these, they challenge the status quo and search for ways to make things happen. They challenge the process, and enable others to do the same.

3. Challenging the process

As an employer, the NHS tends to have difficulty with people who are in favour of real innovation and change. Boat-rocking, stirring, and general disrespect for the status quo is still a sacking offence in many organizations. According to Kouzes and Posner, when leaders challenge the existing order, they do more than overturn a few shibboleths. Their whole purpose is to adventure into unknown places, and act as guides to unfamiliar destinations. Leaders look for opportunities to radically alter, create, revolutionize, and generally shake up systems and people. Before we continue, try Exercise 10.1.

Exercise 10.1 Leaders I have known

- Take a sheet of paper and head it 'Leaders I have known'.
- Draw a line down the middle.
- On the left side, write the names of the leaders who stand out in your mind, irrespective of field, gender, race, age, class, religion, nationality.
- Opposite each name, write the event that you remember them for.

After you have done this, consider the following questions:

- Do any of your leaders have things in common?
- Why do you remember them, and the events you associate them with?
- Did they have particular skills which you believe help to make them memorable?
- Have you tried to emulate any of the people on your list? If so, which ones, and why?
- If these people had not existed, do you believe the events would have happened?

When talking about leaders and leadership, it is easy to forget that what they do is often treated with hostility and met with outrage. When challenged by a leader to become our best, it seems to take too much effort. So we sneer and carp at those who want to set the performance bar a notch higher. We find ways to keep ourselves and others 'just ticking over', doing no more than the minimum required.

Yet the only thing that raises our level of performance, commitment, and motivation is a challenge. Think of how natural disasters pull people together, or how a perceived enemy pushes us to find new ways to win. Leaders are forcing us to recognize that we can do better, and urging us to consider mediocrity unacceptable.

Could it be that acceptance of what leaders do and say is most crucially affected by our perception of our employment status? In *Reinvention of Work: A New Vision of Livelihood for Our Time*, Matthew Fox argues that while 'a job' is about economics, 'work' is how we express our soul, and is unique to all of us. If you think in terms of a job, then the economics are simple – do the job, get paid, and eventually move to another one where the economics are better. But if you have work, then what you do is intrinsically motivating. You still get paid, maybe the same or less than a less-motivated person, but it is much more than a job to you. Leaders have work, not jobs, and they challenge us to have the same (Fox 1994).

Challenging the process creates opportunities for innovation, adventure, stress, and self-development. Operation Raleigh (which offers young people between the ages of 17–23 'the adventure of a lifetime') sums up what leaders do when they challenge the process: 'Venturers Wanted'. Leaders treat every task, project and job as an adventure, an opportunity to create and innovate, especially through other people, and to learn more about themselves. Leaders get the best from others by challenging business-as-usual, and by encouraging the heart.

4. Encouraging the heart

Forgive the language, and acknowledge the intent. Encouraging the heart is primarily about recognizing others' contribution, and celebrating and rewarding successes. Contrast this type of behaviour with what many of us have experienced at work – managers and staff who disparage each other, perceived unfairness in how effort is rewarded, discourtesy, lack of respect, meanness, truculence, grudges, and a general lack of goodwill.

Over the past decade, the NHS has generally become charmless, dispirited, and dull. Increasing workloads and fewer people have left little time for celebrating anything. The near disappearance of the overlap between shifts means there is almost no time to talk to colleagues, share a joke, or gossip. In the search for efficiency we have become ineffective in terms of social relations at work. Add to this the issue of inadequate pay for midwifery, nursing and other groups of staff, and the misery level rises.

But because of the increased stresses, it is even more important to give recognition, and celebrate. A birthday, an anniversary, innovative practice, winning a prize, getting an article published, letters of compliments – anything can trigger a celebration. Let me give you an example. In one unit in which I worked, we finally implemented a patient-held notes scheme after a 2-year hiatus. One lunchtime in the middle of the first week, trays of food appeared – courtesy of the unit's director, celebrating the work of everyone who had contributed to getting the scheme started.

And this was not a 'one off'. We celebrated people, events, services, happy endings, and trying times. We were by no means a perfect unit, but we knew that our contributions were really valued, individually and collectively, and that when we worked hard to make something happen, the effort was noticed.

Ceremonies like the unexpected lunch are important and are not, as many managers like to think, a frivolous waste of time. Far from detracting from efficiency, ceremonies are effective in binding a group and deepening their sense of shared goals.

Kouzes and Posner say that cheerleading and celebrating 'are the processes of honoring people'. This is especially important when monetary rewards are not in the direct remit of the leader. Kouzes and Posner suggest that exemplary leaders can reward, recognize and celebrate volunteers without using money, by:

- *Providing feedback regularly, and not just at the annual appraisal.* We all like to know that we are doing a job well; it helps us to strive harder to improve performance, especially during periods of uncertainty. Imagine if, the first time you tried to walk as a child and fell over, your parents employed the Homer Simpson model of celebrating effort – 'Kids, you tried and failed miserably. The lesson is, never try anything ever again'. There are numerous Homer Simpson-type leaders in the NHS. What we need is more *Star Trek*-type leaders – 'Well done No. 1/Lieutenant/Ensign/alien-life-form-with-ten-tentacles-for-a-head'. Nothing improves performance like on-the-spot praise.
- *Finding people who are doing things right.* In other words, stop the blaming. In any 24-hour day, most of us probably do more things right that we are given credit for. The only way you as a leader will know this is to walk about. If you see the kind of behaviour you want to foster, praise the person on the spot or as soon as possible afterwards – and publicly. You do not have to use purple prose. For example, midwives talk about a colleague being a 'midwives' midwife', but we rarely tell the person concerned. Kouzes and Posner tell of a nursing home in Memphis, Tennessee, where patients often cannot say 'thank you'. So the home recognizes staff with a pin that says 'Caught Caring'. Anyone can give praise on the spot. Do not wait for leaders to do it.
- *Coaching staff.* This is a key part of the performance of any winning team, be it football, athletics, or health care. Coaches focus on what works and how to improve, better, and do differently. Central to coaching are clear values and goals, and linking celebration to these.
- *Creating Pygmalions.*
- *Making recognition public.* Public rewards might cause resentment and jealousy, but private rewards will definitely cause suspicion and charges of favouritism. As a leader, when you demonstrate clearly why you are recognizing an individual or group, you create role models, and prevent feelings of exclusion.
- *Including the people who will benefit from reward systems in designing and monitoring them.*

More than any other fundamental of exemplary leadership, encouraging the heart is closely aligned to culture norms. Leaders and their volunteers in the USA are more at ease with public recognition (there are graduation ceremonies for *kindergarten*), pins and plaques. British workers, generally more reserved (and more accustomed to not being praised?), are less at ease. That is changing, however, with an increasing number of 'praise occasions'. Many are formal (Equality Awards in the NHS, awards in industry and from government departments). But leaders can and must continue to celebrate, reward, and recognize contributions appropriately. We could start by saying 'thank you' to people displaying the kind of behaviours we want to foster. And by having fun at work.

5. Modelling the way

'Practise what you preach'.
'Walk the talk'.
'Put your money where your mouth is'.
'Do what you say you will do'.

These common and maybe clichéd expressions are examples of what leaders must do to model the way. They set the standard and an example for others to follow. Leaders set an example in many ways:

- They focus on values and help others to do the same.
- They encourage dissent in themselves and others.
- They act out their values (behaviour is simply values in action).
- They use calendars, symbols, stories, language, meetings and other tools to show volunteers what is important and what is not.
- They know themselves, and are not afraid to address their faults, vulnerabilities and deficits. They also audit their behaviour.
- They stand up for their beliefs, because they have beliefs to stand for. Remember, if you don't stand for something, you will fall for anything.
- They build small fires. That is, small wins are used to build towards bigger successes. Small fires are more easily tended and are less likely to burn out of control.

Exemplary leaders are a positive force for change and for making a real difference to how organizations and the world in general work. The five fundamentals and their sub-sections presented above are a clear map for any leader who wants to lead in an exemplary manner. I now have to set the opposite side – the cardinal sins of leadership. It is difficult to continue to sin, and continue to be an exemplary leader. Choose.

THE CARDINAL SINS OF LEADERSHIP

I have observed nine fundamental sins of leadership. Some seem minor, others are more toxic. Some you will recognize immediately, others are more insidious and harder to spot. Cumulatively, they can wreck any enterprise.

It's time to put a spotlight on yourself, your organization, and any other venture where you lead are or led; the cardinal sins thrive best in low light, a bit like mushrooms.

Sin 1 – lying to volunteers. This may be an arbitrary sin because many leaders try to protect their followers from what they perceive to be harmful information or news. But if you have stated the facts as you know them, have given people the power to make decisions, and have equipped them with the skills they need to deliver the goals; then protection may actually be self-preservation. Whatever the motive, leaders do not lie to their volunteers, and especially not to protect themselves, financially or otherwise.

Sin 2 – blaming others for your mistakes, failings, or misfortune. This sin is rampant in many organizations, and is particularly virulent in parts of the NHS. It is allied to Sin 3.

Sin 3 – not sharing the gains, and the pain. Recently, the President of the Trades Union Congress called those earning over £50 000 annually, 'greedy bastards' who benefited from all kinds of financial incentives. You may disagree with the words, but recognize the sentiment. In contrast, many low-paid workers receive few perks, are vulnerable to redundancy and consistently receive lower than inflation pay rises. Reward systems in many organizations are unevenly distributed, with senior managers receiving many multiples more in pay and perks than their less financially endowed ·colleagues. Which probably explains why performance related pay has proved to be unpopular – if we work together to achieve goals, why is it that only some people reap the rewards and others are excluded? If the organization fails, why does the pain seem to fall mainly on the followers and not the leaders? Sin 3 concerns how we perceive fairness, justice, and worth.

Sin 4 – abandoning your followers. When the going gets tough, exemplary leaders do not take off in the first life boat. It is not only rats who go down with sinking ships.

Sin 5 – giving up on your followers. I have had leaders tell me that their staff are apathetic, have low morale, have narrow self-interest, and are not competent to do their job. When challenged to say what action they have taken to resolve these problems, a typical answer is 'We sent them on a training course'. Dogs might need training. People do not. Human beings have an instinct for self-improvement, even if not perfectly articulated. To give up on your followers, you have to have first given up on yourself. Sin 5 is evidence of failure of self-belief.

Sin 6 – taking sole credit for the success of your·followers. I have seen so many instances of this that I begin to wonder if the people being sidelined are knowingly giving up recognition of their work. Sin 6 takes many forms – names replaced on reports, names not recorded in minutes of meetings, ideas publicly but skillfully stolen, academic work wrongfully attributed. Followers must take some responsibility for this, and are too often camera-shy and humble. In the few cases where the leader has been found out, they are censured. More often, little or no action is taken. Sin 6 displays a particular set of values about power, accountability, and organizational politics. It is one of the insidious sins which is hard to prove but has a detrimental effect on trust.

Sin 7 – getting carried away by the management or leadership fashion of

the moment. Whether it be management jargon, the latest guru, the hottest theory, or the Number 1 bestseller. Make up your own mind. Better still, write your own jargon, bestseller or theory. Whatever you are thinking about leadership, so are millions of others. It's just that your framework or context is different. Plough your own furrow.

Sin 8 – undermining your followers, spreading rumours about them, or gossiping about them to others. (Unless it is to publicly praise and celebrate their achievements.) This sin is also insidious. It is prevalent in organizations, and hard to resist. It is also destructive of trust, loyalty, friendship and love. Sin 8 primarily serves to distance a leader from followers they believe will hinder their future success.

Sin 9 – not knowing you have sinned. Lack of insight and hubris are the primary causes of Sin 9.

This list of Cardinal Sins is not exhaustive. You have your own. But you must begin to notice and correct the behaviour that prevents you from becoming an exemplary leader.

Writing this book has revealed my own sins, and it has not always been pleasant. But growing as a leader demands more than reading a few books, attending a course or two and listening to the gurus expound. Growing into a leader is a journey, and at each stage you find a place on the map that you have missed or did not know was there. Exemplary leaders are not sin-free. They simply accept the sin, forgive the sinner, and correct the behaviour. Simply?

THE FIVE FUNDAMENTAL PRACTICES (Kouzes and Posner 1995)

- Inspiring a Shared Vision
- Enabling Others to Act
- Challenging the Process
- Encouraging the Heart
- Modelling the Way

THE 10 COMMITTMENTS OF LEADERSHIP (Kouzes and Posner 1995)

- Enlist others
- Envision the future
- Strengthen others
- Foster collaboration
- Search for opportunities
- Experiment and take risks
- Celebrate and cheer accomplishments
- Recognize contributions

- Set the example
- Achieve small wins

Key learning point

- You cannot be an exemplary leader and expect to keep on sinning with no consequences.

REFERENCES

Bass B M, Avolio B J 1994 Shatter the glass ceiling: women may make better managers. Human Resource Management 33(4): 549–560
Fox M 1994 Reinvention of work: a new vision of livelihood for our time. Harper San Francisco, San Francisco
Kouzes J M, Posner B M 1995 The leadership challenge: how to keep getting extraordinary things done in organizations. Jossey-Bass, San Francisco

Nurse leaders for the 21st century

Key words:

balance of responsibilities; diversity; demographics; nurse education; collaboration and partnerships; community participation; skills to survive and grow; barriers to achieving leadership

Current research on leadership focuses on the need for tomorrow's leaders to be team players. The literature, particularly that relating to how women lead, stresses cooperative models of working, such as 'post-heroic transformational leadership' as defined by Bradford and Cohen (1984).

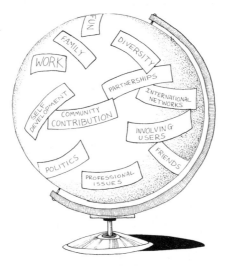

Future leader

Effective leaders are not stand-alone heroes, but work in cooperative ways with others. Traditional 'fixed' styles of leadership, based on reward or punishment, continue to give way to 'situational leadership', where the leader has regard for both people *and* process, and action depends on the situation being faced. In health services, Stewart urges leaders to be aware of the need for 'external leadership', touching those points in the organization's environment which have an impact on its operations and its values (Stewart 1988). With specific reference to community health workers, Wilkinson shows how this group, mainly women, had a significant impact on Black-American communities from the 1960s onwards (Wilkinson 1992).

Nurses, both as healthcare workers and as citizens, have a significant leadership role in how healthcare services are planned and delivered. The 1979 WHO Alma Ata Declaration (Health for All 2000) clearly outlined the role of the nurse in enabling communities to achieve improved health status. Continuing initiatives worldwide to involve communities in planning and delivering health services have created a need for healthcare organizations to find alternatives to the command and control style of management.

The NHS, however, still actively portrays this discredited style of management, exemplified in the treatment it metes out to so-called 'whistle blowers' – staff who turn to alternative sources of support (such as the media) to bolster their campaigns to promote patient care, or expose irregularities in clinical or financial management. Management's attempts to keep people in their place is clearly at odds with the need to collaborate and form partnerships with a multitude of groups and organizations who may have very diverse, but valid, views of health and health care.

The leadership and vision needed to keep developing the NHS is lacking at many levels, and barriers which inhibit the leadership potential of nurses have been imposed. Nazarko has identified four fronts on which nurse leaders are inhibited within the nursing home sector (Nazarko 1996):

1. Pressure of work, which has seen a particularly steep increase over the last 3 years.
2. Lack of support for leaders and little commitment to their development.
3. Disunity and lack of clear goals within the sector.
4. Financial constraints, which impact on funds for training.

I would argue that these four barriers, and more, also exist within the acute and community hospital sectors. There is little evidence that they will substantially decrease in the foreseeable future. We have to lead in spite of them, and find solutions as we go along.

Nurses need alternative ways of thinking about what we do, who we do it with, why we do it, and how we do it. The NHS has been lazy and complacent about preparing healthcare leaders for the 21st century, leaving healthcare workers and the communities they work with feeling frustrated, mistrustful of each other, and disillusioned. Nurses need a much wider preparation. Placing nurse education in universities is a positive step, but universities are not always inclined to teach and encourage innovative leadership theory nor, indeed, have they always been inspirational role models in how to enact leadership principles. Having university-educated nurses will not by itself create the nurse leaders we need. That takes something else – an understanding of what nurses might be, and can be, over the next 50 or so years.

What challenges do nurse leaders of the future face? How will we be led in the growing chaos that is affecting health care, and how will we lead?

SEARCHING FOR THE NEW LAMPLIGHTERS

I believe there are five main challenges that nurse leaders of the future face:

1. Defining and understanding leadership
2. Working with non-organizational leaders
3. The provision of care
4. Workforce issues
5. High technology and low care?

Defining and understanding leadership

In one of his editorials in *Nursing Management*, Tom Keighley makes it clear that for the foreseeable future 'the journal will focus on leadership in nursing and health care'. (Keighley 1996). This is very welcome, but leadership has not been high on nurses' agendas as a topic of study, nor have nurses taken leadership skills seriously enough.

Sams, writing about her personal experience of participating in a programme on leadership skills for community nurses, argues that while leadership skills are intrinsic to nursing practice, 'these skills are often underrated, and sometimes unrecognized by practitioners themselves' (Sams 1996). A speaker at a nursing conference in the UK argued that student nurses complete their training without learning to become team players, or leaders (Casey 1996).

But if we have been tardy in recognizing the need to understand and define leadership and what it means for nursing in the past, we are making up for lost time. The Royal College of Nursing (RCN), for instance, has a management forum whose newsletter is called, simply, *Leader*, and has launched and directed the Ward Leadership project I have referred to earlier in the book. The King's Fund also runs a leadership programme (for potential nurse directors).

Since the mid-1990s, there has been a mini-explosion in writings on leadership appearing in the nursing and healthcare press, here and abroad (for example, Antrobus 1998, Bowman 1997, Casey 1995, Cunningham &

Whitby 1997, Falco Scott 1995, Girvin 1996, Greenwood 1997, Malby 1996, Nazarko 1996, Rafferty 1996, RCN Nursing Update Unit 062 1995, Wedderburn Tate 1996b). But why has it taken so long for nurses in the UK to become interested in the concept of leadership, and acknowledge their responsibilities as healthcare leaders?

Part of the explanation for this may lie in the way many people still equate management with leadership. Nurses have a historic mistrust of managers, which may have affected their understandings and opinions of leadership. Yet management and leadership are different things, as I hope this book has shown. Kotter argues that the thing we call 'management' is a product of the strict conditions of the last 100 years or so, in which we have seen the advent of mass production, global capitalism and the worldwide economy. Leadership, on the other hand, is ageless (Kotter 1990). Kotter summarizes leadership as 'movement', and management as 'consistency and order'. Both types of behaviour are needed for the effectiveness of any project, but their specific focus is different, and they give different results. Table 11.1 summarizes these concepts.

Table 11.1 Leadership or management? (Adapted from Kotter 1990)

Leadership	Management
Aligns people into teams, and coalitions	Staff and structure, policies and procedures
Sets direction	Plans and budgets
Focuses on change	Predictability and order
Motivates, inspires	Problem-solving and control
	Energizes

Nurses will derive great benefit from striving to understand the differences between management and leadership, and by consequence, the differences between managers and leaders. Without such understanding, we will not be able to fully realize our potential as leaders. Nor will we be able to recognize leaders in non-corporate/organizational settings.

Working with non-organizational leaders

As the delivery of health care continues to shift from hospital to community, nurses of the future will need to employ different types of leadership skill when working with patients, families and communities. It would be prudent, therefore, to include the study of non-corporate models of leadership in the preparation of nurses.

I first became conscious of non-corporate forms of leadership when I worked on community-focused, and community-led, healthcare projects in the USA. Since then I have realized that there are several examples of this type of leadership in the UK (Wedderburn Tate 1996a, Mawson 1998). Non-corporate forms of leadership exist in most community groups, and are beginning to interest some organizations (DePree 1997). Box 11.1 outlines some of the characteristics of non-corporate forms of leadership as I have observed them.

Box 11.1   Some characteristics of non-corporate forms of leadership

- No formal leaders (leaders emerge out of events)
- A lack of formality between leader and followers
- Leaders depend on personal power (influence), not resource and position power
- Leadership role changes hands on several occasions
- Confusion, factionalism, and divided loyalties
- Leaders tend to be more charismatic
- Few structures or procedures

Such characteristics pose problems for those more accustomed to the conventional boundaries within which formal leaders work. This is already a contentious issue for the NHS and other statutory organizations (local authority, the Civil Service, and others) who are now contracting increasingly commonly with community agencies led by non-corporate leaders. Tensions are being experienced on both sides: by non-corporate leaders who, for example, find the way issues such as accountability are addressed by formal organizations restrictive; and by formal leaders, who are perhaps uncomfortable about the casual approach of non-formal leaders to issues such as bureaucratic structures.

In Chapter 12, I will offer examples of some of the consequences of this tension. For the moment, the important thing is that nurses are aware that there are different forms of leadership. Nurses of the future need to be able to adapt their preferred leadership style when working with an increasingly diverse range of patients and communities, and they should be exposed to alternative models of leadership from early in their basic education curriculum. The evidence to date, however, suggests that little attention is being given to this issue in the education sector. The preparation of nurses for leadership is neither systematic nor sufficiently broad to take account of non-corporate models of leadership. Yet the third challenge we face demands such preparation.

The provision of care

Increasing concentration on reducing the cost of healthcare provision has created an ongoing debate about who gets what, when, and how. Despite our reluctance to recognize it as such, there is really only one name for this activity – rationing.

Rationing has been an underlying tension in the NHS throughout its life (Goodman 1998). As we continue to evade the moral and other arguments that surround rationing, the increasing fragmentation of healthcare provision occurs without clearly defined parameters. Having diverse provision of health care is entirely appropriate; but without clearly prescribed boundaries, monitoring of the quality of care is difficult.

Like most countries, the UK has a mixed economy of healthcare provision. Unlike many, however, we seem to have a deep-seated resistance to private and voluntary sector involvement. But we have to recognize that the NHS cannot do it all. The needs of different communities and particular groups of people in our increasingly cosmopolitan society require variety and diversity in the healthcare services on offer. The input of private and voluntary organizations, and of individuals and communities, are likely to assume even greater prominence as we move into the 21st century.

Nurses have a key role to play in preventing vulnerable groups from being excluded from healthcare policy. Concerted attempts to involve the public in how health care is planned and delivered will be instrumental in getting difficult and controversial issues such as rationing onto the table for public debate. But the general citizenry's involvement in healthcare planning and delivery may be a two-edged sword. Numerous surveys suggest that while 'the public' would defend the NHS to the death, they want to see it spend most of its money on the health of children and people who can contribute to the economy. This inevitably leads to questions of equity, fairness, and accountability, and about the efficacy of the 'citizens' juries' who look as though they might become key players in the decisions governing the provision of health care.

How far should a jury of citizens influence key decisions about what to spend on health care, and where? In the past few years, there have been examples of how 'ordinary people' view such issues as heart surgery for smokers (do not deserve it), health care for people with HIV and AIDS (do not deserve it), and IVF (ambivalent). Understandings of the needs of people with physical, sensory and mental disabilities are still shrouded in ignorance. On the other hand, public outrage has caused reviews and even reversals of decisions taken in splendid isolation by health boards or trusts, such as the policy of some hospitals to restrict access to heart surgery and stroke services to people over a certain age.

Healthcare professionals who front the NHS need to talk with each other about our priorities for our communities, and we also need to educate the wider public about the realities of healthcare funding, provision, and outcomes. We have to push ideas like the NHS is not free, we cannot live forever, technology cannot solve all our ills, children die, and older people benefit in similar ways to younger people from all types of medical and surgical interventions.

Providing the care populations need depends upon having the physical capacity to deliver that care. In this area, nursing is facing a real crisis. The declining numbers of qualified nurses, midwives and health visitors is a potential disaster for nurses and nursing.

Workforce issues

Nursing shortages need to be seen in the context of general employment trends. Across Europe, there are approximately 21 million unemployed people, with the relatively prosperous Northern Europe (which includes the UK) having less unemployment than the economically poorer south. Unemployment is highest among young people, and where there are jobs, employers prefer to endorse over-time for full-time workers rather than use job-shares or have more flexible work times. Where flexible work shifts do exist, they tend to focus on poorly paid part-time jobs for women, with few career prospects.

NHS Trusts tend to follow this rigid pattern of seeing full-time work as the norm, with few alternatives being offered. But trusts are now recognizing that nurses' skills are in demand by a range of employers, not just those in health care, and the NHS's reputation as an inflexible, bureaucratic, hierarchical, slow-moving organization does not always make it the employer of choice. This, combined with causes outlined below, means the health service suffers recurring nurse shortages of varying degrees of magnitude.

Over the past decade and a half, there has been a steady decline in the number of entrants to pre-registration nursing courses. In 1984, there were 75 000 pupils and student nurses in England; by 1994, the number had been reduced by more than 50%. There are several explanations for this, including:

- a narrow focus on 17-year-old school leavers as the main entrants
- increased entry qualifications (through Project 2000)
- poor pay
- lack of integrated workforce planning
- better opportunities on offer elsewhere
- racialism (against black and minority ethnic groups)
- the discontinuation of enrolled nurse training.

If getting nurses into training is a problem, so is retaining them after qualification. For a major employer, the NHS is spectacularly bad at ensuring that it has the people to deliver the service. Since the 1990 reforms, both Trusts and the Department of Health have taken a narrow view of nursing numbers, mainly to limit the pay bill of the NHS. This has been exacerbated by two factors:

1. The implementation of Project 2000, which reduced the amount of time nurse students spend delivering direct care.

2. The economic recession in the early 1990s, which decreased nurses' mobility and therefore reduced nursing vacancies.

With the economic upturn in the mid-1990s, Trusts continued to make parochial assessments of how many qualified nurses they needed. These numbers were always moving down, with the gaps being plugged by the appointment of new healthcare assistants. Meanwhile, the Department of Health's 'light touch' management of Trusts meant that central planning of the NHS workforce fell into neglect. The culmination of this cost-containment approach to nurse recruitment and retention is yet another cycle of nurse shortages.

Shortage of nurses is not a new phenomenon. Between 1932 and 1972, there were at least four major reports on nursing shortages, three of which predated the existence of the NHS (see Box 11.2). Depressingly, however, few of the major recommendations of these reports, or those of more recent times, have been enacted. The majority of trusts, for instance, do not have annualized hours which enable managers to match available nursing time to care over a whole year. Neither do they have systematic ways of ensuring that nurses take career breaks, and that nurses on maternity leave are kept in touch with their employers. Nor did Trusts anticipate the huge demand for nurses that resulted from the growth of nursing homes, both private and local authority.

Box 11.2 Major reports on nursing shortages (Buchan 1998)

1932 – The Lancet Commission on Nursing
Focus – rates of nursing vacancies.
Recommendations – provision of in-service training, better pay, reform nurse education, and more domestic staff.
1939 – The Interdepartmental Committee on Nursing Services (Interim Report, Ministry of Health)
Focus – shortage of staff nurses.
Recommendations – reform of nurse education, more ward orderlies, employ more married nurses, and national pensions and salaries.
1947 – Report of the Ministry of Health Working Party on the Recruitment and Training of Nurses
Focus – the continued nursing shortage.
Recommendations – more male nurses, no restriction on married nurses staying in post, more part-time employment, and all nurse students to have full student status.
1972 – The Briggs Report (proper title: report of the Committee on Nursing)
Focus – nurse shortages, especially in care of the elderly and psychiatry. This report also stressed the importance of identifying healthcare needs before correcting shortages.
Recommendations – many of the above plus, more mature entrants, create a scheme for nurses who want to return to the NHS, keep in touch with nurses on maternity leave, and allocate staff according to workload. The Briggs report is most famous for its emphasis on nursing becoming a graduate profession.

The Department of Health has belatedly tried to get back into a position where it can have an influence over nurse recruitment through advertising campaigns and other publicity activities, but these are unlikely to provide longterm solutions to nurse shortages. A favoured tactic of trust managers – recruiting nurses from overseas – is also unlikely to provide the answers. The UK has a very chequered history of welcoming overseas recruits in time of crisis, then rejecting them in times of plenty. Continuing to depend on overseas recruitment to solve nursing shortages increases complacency and absolves managers of the responsibility of seeking lasting, longterm solutions. And taking nurses from the Philippines or elsewhere simply shifts the shortage to another country.

The challenge facing nurse leaders is to find longterm solutions to nursing shortages. Locally, we can start by being more visible in our communities. What is the image of nursing and nurses in your local community? We also need to improve working conditions in our organizations. It is ironic that when we most need to have *more* alternatives to full-time working, many Trusts are employing a single approach – short-term contracts – and do so not to boost recruitment, but to cut costs. 'Return to nursing' schemes and nursing refresher courses are also affected by this narrow focus on reducing wage costs.

Nationally, we can look again at the recommendations in past reports which addressed nursing shortages and influenced policy makers to think more broadly about workforce planning. A better national oversight of the UK labour market as a whole, and nursing in particular, linked to a capacity within trusts and other NHS providers to apply workforce planning methods would create a more systematic approach to managing nurse shortages.

High technology and low care?

On an everyday level in health care, technology is taken for granted. Computerized laboratory results, beds that are raised and lowered by the touch of a foot, cardiac monitoring (babies and adults), ventilators, dimmer switches, telephone networks, word processing, record storage, electronic mail, infusion pumps – all are so familiar that their absence or dysfunction can disrupt our day, and patients' lives.

Technology has also increased the availability of information, including health information. Anyone with access to the Internet can, in a few seconds, be connected to any library in the world, and access any information available on that system. But, as with health care itself, millions of people have no access to this resource. The growing gap between the informed rich and the uninformed poor, at least as defined by access to high technology, may create healthcare problems associated with disenfranchisement, lack of control over healthcare interventions and social isolation and exclusion.

The growth of telemedicine (providing health care at a distance from patients) is a major challenge for nurses, who place great value on the emotional, face-to-face aspects of health care. One project shows we can have it all. The Telemedicine Group at Edinburgh University leads a project which enables women to receive specialist ante-natal care at home (Clark 1996). Midwives linked to a maternity hospital database can perform cardiotocography (CTG) and monitor a woman's blood pressure in the comfort of her own home. The Edinburgh scheme is part of a Europe-wide project on telemedicine. Similar projects exist in the USA (some centrally funded), and in remote areas of Canada where access to hospital can be difficult.

Telemedicine may reduce the costs of in-patient treatment, while improving access to specialist services, but the biggest advantage is the reduced need to uproot patients from their locality to receive specialist treatment. This places the patient, not the practitioner, at the centre of the consultation, and may also improve the relationship between a range of practitioners by helping them to share experiences and skills more widely.

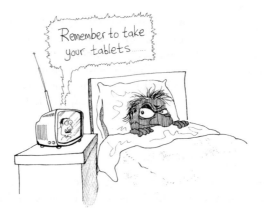

Telemedicine

If nurse leaders are to survive in this future, what skills, knowledge, and behaviours will they need?

LEADING THE FUTURE

I believe that nurses must develop an effective range of skills in the following areas:

- lobbying
- political leadership
- policy analysis

- facilitation
- negotiation
- networking
- building multi-sector alliances
- community development
- crap detecting.

Not all nurses will need all these skills all of time, but they need to be acquired by a wide range of nurse leaders. There are many ways of acquiring them. One is through the leadership projects mentioned above. Other methods include activity within our professional organizations, consulting with colleagues and our local communities, mentoring, and through personal and strategic networks.

We need to acquire the skills in three contexts:

1. Knowledge (knowing that, knowing how, knowing beyond/the future).
2. Effective processes (negotiating, networking, enabling, including coaching).
3. Tasks (identify, select/prioritize, implement, evaluate).

Leaders succeed when they are consistently effective on all fronts. If the list seems daunting, consider what has happened to nursing in the latest restructuring of the NHS – the formation of primary care groups. Once again we appear to be on the outside, hoping that our absence will be noticed and we will be invited to join in the revolution/evolution. Nurse leaders must start now to change the perception of nurses as 'nice, kind people' who keep a low profile and prefer not to engage in politics. Which brings me to crap detecting.

Active crap detectors are vital if nurses are to have any lasting influence on health policy. We need to stand back, think, reflect, and call it as we see it. We cannot afford to stick our heads in the sand and hope that, if we keep quiet (as we have done), someone else will solve our problems. If we are to succeed with leadership, we need to act like leaders. We may have to become unpopular in the process, nuisances, raging champions for change, and be generally less liked than we have tended to be. We need to challenge ourselves and each other to want to create a different way of working with our colleagues, communities and with governments. Collaboration and cooperation, health, community enabling, leadership, and effective systems and practices are our focus.

As a starting point, to challenge yourself, take a moment to consider the questions in Exercise 11.1. You can add to the list, and share them with your colleagues.

Exercise 11.1   If not me, who?

- What is my primary role as a leader?

- How can I contribute to healthcare policy?
- What skills will I need to meet my objectives as a leader?
- How many ways can a leader lead?
- What obstacles are there to my leading?
- Who can I collaborate with to meet my objectives as a leader?

To succeed consistently, nurse (and healthcare) leaders of the future will need to challenge themselves more often than at present. By having a better understanding of leadership and how it differs from management, we will be more able to choose to lead. Knowing more about alternatives to corporate forms of leadership will enhance our capacity to work with a wide range of health and social care providers led by people who do it differently. These experiences will enable us to be less introverted, more outward-looking, and less likely to dismiss what is different as of little or no importance to us.

By leading without power, we release the potential in our followers, and the development potential within ourselves. By accepting our leadership role in health care, and as citizens, nursing is more likely to survive another millennium.

Key learning points

- Nurses must lead, in spite of barriers.
- Nursing shortages are amenable to longterm solutions.
- Leaders do it without power.
- Nurse leaders of the future need a wide range of skills, including crap detecting.

REFERENCES

Antrobus S 1998 Political leadership in nursing. Nursing Management 5(4): 26–28
Bowman G 1997 Over managed. Nursing Standard 11(19): 24–25
Bradford D L, Cohen A R 1984 Managing for excellence, Wiley, Chichester
Buchan J 1998 Your country needs you. Health Service Journal 108(5613): 22–25
Casey N 1995 The great quest for leadership. Nursing Standard 10(12–14): 49–52
Casey N 1996 Student nurses unable to provide leadership. Nursing Standard 11(8): 8
Clark G 1996 On-line midwives. Nursing Times 92(3): 18–19
Cunningham G, Whitby E 1997 Power redistribution. Health Management, September: 14–15
DePree M 1997 Leading without power: finding hope in serving community. Jossey-Bass, San Francisco
Falco Scott F 1995 Getting to the Year 2000. Caring, October: 17–18
Girvin J 1996 Leadership and nursing: Part 1: history and politics. Nursing Management 3(1): 10–12

Goodman M 1998 Ethical issues in health care rationing. Nursing Management 29–33

Greenwood A 1997 Leadership for change. Nursing Standard 11(19): 22–24

Keighley T 1996 Editorial. Nursing Management 2(9): 3

Kotter J P 1990 A force for change: how leadership differs from management. The Free Press, London

Malby R 1996 King's Fund ignites the lights. Nursing Management 2(8): 11–13

Mawson A 1998 The rise of the social entrepreneur. Journal of the Royal Society of Arts cxlv(5484); 1/4, 91–99

Nazarko L 1996 Home front leadership. Nursing Management 3(1): 16–17

Rafferty A-M 1996 Political leadership in nursing: the role of nursing in health care reform. Final Harkness Report (Commonwealth Fund of New York). Unpublished.

RCN Nursing Update, Unit 062 1995 Leadership in nursing: more than one way. Nursing Standard 13(10)

Sams D 1996 The development of leadership skills in clinical practice. Nursing Times 96(28): 37–39

Stewart R 1988 Leading in the NHS: a practical guide. Macmillan, London

Wedderburn Tate C 1996b Different ways to make a difference. Nursing Standard 10(29): 20

Wedderburn Tate C 1996a Out of the trench: developing nurse leaders. Nursing Standard 10(24): supplement, 8–9

Wilkinson D Y 1992 Indigenous community health workers in the 1960s and beyond. In: Braithwaite R L, Taylor SE (eds) Health issues in the black community. Jossey-Bass, San Francisco

Diverse leaders: non-corporate models of leadership

Key words:

difference; non-corporate; community development; volunteers;
leadership styles

So far, our exploration has centred on leadership as it is practised (or not) in formal organizations. In Chapter 11, I introduced the idea that there are other forms of leadership which equally deserve our attention. At least one leader of a major company in the USA has used such a model (De Pree 1997). Alternative forms of leadership do exist, they have just not been studied in as much detail as the more traditional forms.

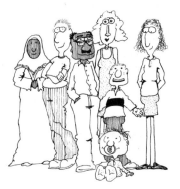

Diversity in leadership

In this chapter, I want to explore alternative forms of leadership, and consider how they can add to our understanding of leaders and leadership.

As we move through the ideas, I want you to think about those parts of your organization which appear to be led differently from the norm, either because of what needs to be done or how the leaders behave.

I will use stories to illustrate how I believe non-corporate leaders differ from their corporate counterparts. You may recognize yourself as one of these different types of leaders, as well as making connections with the transformational aspects of leadership we talked about before. I hope that our journey will help both of us to think, talk and act differently about leaders and leadership.

NON-CORPORATE, STILL A LEADER

My first consciousness about the existence of non-corporate forms of leadership was sparked by the year I spent working with a non-profit agency (the US term for a voluntary sector organization) in New York City in 1992. The agency's main activities at the time centred on initiatives to reduce the high levels of perinatal deaths in its locality. I will talk more about this later. For now, suffice to say that this agency was more than an organization, a word whose meanings include 'ordered' and 'structured'. There were all the normal tensions you would expect to find in any workplace, but there was also an excitement about the work that was being done.

At about the same time as it began to dawn on people that there were probably other types of leaders and leadership than the corporate norm, writings and research on leadership began to focus more on transformational leadership, looking at leaders who care about people as well as the 'bottom line', leaders who inspire, motivate, and mobilize followers on whom they are dependent. Much of this research was engendered by the obvious leadership deficits in the structured organizations where many people made their living. These deficits included lack of inspiration and imagination, low motivation and innovation, poor development of people's potential, and general apathy and cynicism. It was not all bad news, but something was obviously seriously wrong with structured organizations worldwide.

I saw similar behaviour in many parts of the NHS, other agencies I was working with, and in the voluntary sector. It therefore seemed strange to me that voluntary sector leadership was not the focus of more attention and interest from researchers on leadership. This place where many of the transformational aspects of leadership were clearly (but quietly) visible, remained unexplored.

In the UK, the voluntary sector was increasing in size, and was becoming more involved in providing the services the government was opting out from. Leadership of this sector was therefore important if clients were to receive benefit from the change of provider. My working life encompassed both the NHS and the voluntary sector. I served two voluntary agencies, one concerned with health, the other with young people. I therefore experienced at first hand, the differences in how both sectors viewed leadership.

Both of the voluntary sector agencies I served receive funding from the NHS. A major cause of frustration for us was the slow response of funders to changes in our clients' needs, and to our need for clarity on funders' yearly intentions. The closure of the agency providing health care was partly attributable to this. The agency for young people experiences similar frustrations, but these stem from the stultifying rate at which local government operates, and the inevitable incursions of politics.

I used to think that the statutory sector simply did not understand how voluntary groups operated, but I become more convinced each day that the heart of the issue is that both sectors view the work they have to do very differently. For example, in the voluntary sector, if targets are not met, funding is withdrawn. Voluntary sector staff are therefore much more driven to achieve what they set out to do. Furthermore, they choose a particular agency because they believe in what it stands for. I am not saying that people who work in structured organizations do not believe in what they do; I am saying that in the non-corporate sector, everyone is clear on how what they do affects the health and survival of the whole. If staff in an agency do not perform, funding goes, and so does their job.

Think of the NHS. People get paid every month, no questions asked. Even though the 1991 reforms mean that hospitals can be closed, such decisions are usually driven by financial constraints, not the quality of care. There appears to be a lack of urgency about many things in the NHS – poor care, waiting lists, complaints, racialism, information systems, leadership, staff development, justice, industrial relations. It is almost impossible to lose your job in a large organization unless you (finally) kill somebody, waste money, or have sex with your patient (or student). In the meantime, you can mistreat clients, give poor quality service, hinder colleagues, fail to meet agreed objectives, do not believe in what you are doing, fail to lead, neglect accountability, and still pass go to a pay cheque. Inspiration, mobilization, motivation, and leadership dependency appear to count for little.

In *Leading Without Power*, Max De Pree argues that what is needed in our world is more 'movements' as opposed to more organizations (as in 'structured' and 'ordered') (De Pree 1997). He describes a movement as an 'exceptional organization', 'a collective state of mind, a public and common understanding that the future can be created, not simply experienced or endured'. De Pree's exemplars of such organizations are non-profit groups (the voluntary sector) in the USA, but in my experience (my above spleen-venting notwithstanding), this phenomenon also exists in structured organizations in the public and private sectors.

Movements are characterized as having (De Pree 1997):

- harmonious relationships

- constructive conflict
- palpable unity in pursuing the agreed vision
- innovation
- a sense of urgency
- high levels of trust.

Have you ever worked in a organization like that? Maybe the immediate group of people with whom you work has some of these characteristics, especially if you have been together for several years. Maybe the above characteristics extend to the department in which you are based. But would it describe the whole organization, a word whose meanings include 'orderly and structured'? Probably not, because size tends to slow many of the processes which enable exceptional organizations.

With an entity the size of the NHS, we would have to look at the micro level to find anything resembling a movement as described by De Pree, examples of which include the Apple computer company in its early years, and the Beth Israel Hospital in Boston (a colleague who had worked at Beth Israel always spoke of the unique experience she had, and longed to return). Apple Computers grew, became an organization, and then lost momentum and direction. Beth Israel seems to be an ironic exception. A hospital must be one of the most structured of workplaces, but Beth Israel seems able to offer the best of both worlds – order and spontaneity, structure and innovation, leadership and management.

Before we go much further, it would be a good idea to say something about Max De Pree. What is his evidence for the existence of exceptional organizations where people are inspired, motivated, and mobilized to achieve?

Max De Pree is a past Chief Executive of Herman Miller, Inc., a very successful family-owned furniture manufacturer based in Michigan. From his writings, De Pree appears to have strong Christian beliefs, which might explain his firm conviction that leaders are the servants of their followers. This belief and concepts such as integrity, tolerance and grace imbued his leadership of both Herman Miller, and the non-profit organizations he serves.

Herman Miller pioneered the concept of work teams, of which there were initially 350, with 4 to 25 people in a team. Now with nearly 7000 employees, they still use work teams, but have adapted the concept so as not to lose the sense of community they had at the beginning. Herman Miller also invented the Scanlon Plan in 1952, a scheme whereby workers gain financially from the results of their suggestions for improved productivity. Versions of the Scanlon Plan are now common in many US companies.

Since 1983, Herman Miller has been on the list of the *100 Best Companies to Work for in America*. This is a yearly independent survey of US companies (the top 10 in 1997 included Microsoft and Hewlett Packard, both exceptional organizations). *Fortune*, the capitalist's capitalist business magazine, named Herman Miller as one of the 10 best-managed and most innovative companies in the USA. Herman is also a Fortune 500 company (that is, one of 500 companies which are deemed the most successful in terms of sales, return on investment and other criteria.) It might be useful to consider some of Herman Miller's vital statistics (from 1996) which are listed in Box 12.1.

Box 12.1   Herman Miller, Inc. (Fisher et al 1998)

Founded   1923
Total number of employees   6798
Staff turnover   6%
Applications received   6000
New jobs created over 2 years   433
Revenues   £1.5 billion
Fortune 500 ranking   456
Rank according to longterm return on investment   Seventh
Focus   People and profits

So this is no fly-by-night company. It just does things differently, and successfully. For example, one famous Herman Miller product is the Eames chair (created by the great American designer, Charles Eames), made from moulded fibreglass. The company knew the chair would sell but had no money to buy a piece of equipment to produce it. One of the regional sales managers loaned the company the money, the chair was produced and became a best-seller.

Herman Miller operates many organizations under one umbrella. They must be doing something right if the company has been consistently profitable, and ranks in the top 10 over a 10-year period for return on investment (the 'bottom line'). Herman Miller is not an aberration. The edge they have is leadership of the transformational variety, on the non-corporate model.

The exceptional organizations I have observed have the characteristics outlined in Box 12.2.

These groups also tend to focus on only a few issues, are quick to respond to opportunities as well as threats, and are very civil to each other (even when having heated debates).

A closer look reveals that leadership in such groups is more untidy, more spontaneous, and is available to everyone. Formal meetings (ones with agendas), if they are held, are led by the person who volunteered, not by the most senior person in the room at the time. The role of leader is fluid, each person taking the role as appropriate. This can (and does) lead to friction within the organization, but more often than not, such friction is out in the open. Emotions are closer to the surface and are more immediate.

Box 12.2 Exceptions to the rule

- Mainly, but not exclusively, in the voluntary sector.
- Significant numbers of women take leadership roles.
- Passionate and intense about the work to be done.
- Non-hierarchical, and are wary of bureaucratic procedures.
- Take risks, and expect to make mistakes.
- Express emotion (anger, hostility, fear) openly, and regard this as healthy.
- Competence (technical and relational) is highly rated.
- Staff are markedly more diverse than in a standard organization.
- Leaders overflowing with ideas that drive the vision.
- Leaders are no more or less charismatic than other leaders.
- Development (people, services, processes) is a key priority.
- People have fun at work.

Such behaviour may frighten those of us who have become used to plans being made and not completed, inured to being disappointed by leaders who do not keep their word, and who are generally cynical about 'bosses'. The leaders on exceptional organizations are not bosses, but they're not saints either. What they have is an unshakable faith in the capacity of their followers, on whom they are dependent, and who they treat as volunteers.

It may not be surprising that non-corporate forms of leadership exist in the voluntary sector. After all, volunteers do not get paid, so something else must be driving them. De Pree argues that movements are driven by love – love of the work being done, of the people for each other, and of the satisfaction of producing the best results they can. Probably the most appropriate analogy for this is a family.

We have, hopefully, all had at least one experience when the work we were doing, and the people we were working with, produced such a high, that it lives in our memory. If you think about group dynamics, movements are the 'performing' stage of that process. At each stage of a group's development, the leader plays a different role (Box 12.3).

Box 12.3 Stages of group dynamics (Adapted from Blanchard 1996)

Stage 1 – The group is trying to orient itself to the task and to each other. The group leader's role is primarily *directive*.
Stage 2 – The group begins to settle down, but friction and conflict exist around the leader's authority, and uncertainty about her or his competence arises. The group leader's role is that of a coach, a balance between *direction* and *support*.
Stage 3 – The group is more sure of itself, conflict is reduced, goals are being met, and other leaders are emerging. The group leader's role is primarily *supportive*. Direction is given only if a new task is presented to the group.
Stage 4 – The group is performing well, and are supportive and caring of each other. Emergent leaders are encouraged to develop their skills. The group leader's role is to provide *support* and *direction* as needed. The emphasis is on delegation.

In the groups I have watched going through these stages, Stage 3 happens so quickly that it may be missed. Think of a group you belong or belonged to, one that had a high level of energy and performance. Can you pin-point when you stopped fighting each other and started working together? If the group leader is skilled in recognizing the development stages, Stage 3 is barely noticed. Non-corporate leaders seem very adept at this, probably because they acknowledge that they experience the same anxieties, frustrations, and ultimate joy as the rest of the group.

The distance between leaders and followers in non-corporate organizations is much less because there are fewer layers of people, and little hierarchy. There is more informality. This is the starkest difference I notice between how I lead in the voluntary sector organization I serve, and the leadership positions I held in the NHS. I also serve as a volunteer with a community Trust, which generally acts more like the voluntary sector group than the regional health authority (RHA). Maybe size does count. But more than that, it is how small groups of committed people respond to their environment that marks out the non-corporate forms of leadership. Let me give you an example from the voluntary sector agency in the USA that I served.

One of the agency's major projects (more details below) was funded by the federal government (that is, the Congress). Mid-way through the project, it was clear that the fundraising plan had to be updated. While this was in preparation, a major funder, based in Washington DC, invited the agency to a presentation about their funding priorities for the year.

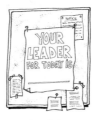

Flexibility

The event was on a Thursday. The invitation arrived 2 days before. The agency's fund raiser was backed up with work for the next week and had no time. You would assume that the chief executive would make the trip in her place. Not so. The agency's representative to the presentation in Washington was a local resident who had been a volunteer with the agency for several years. She knew their work, their philosophy, and their funding needs, and she was delegated the authority to make agreements with the Washington funder on behalf of the agency.

What I found interesting about this process was the reaction of the agency's local funders (the city and state governments). They strongly disapproved of the agency's action, even though 'involving local residents in the work of the community-based agencies' was a key part of their operating philosophy. The competence of the person was not in doubt; position appeared to be the over-riding criterion for attendance at the meeting in Washington.

I want to try now to summarize our discussion so far by showing how I think non-corporate organizations and their leaders differ from their corporate counterparts. First, the differences between the two types of leader.

Table 12.1   Different strokes

Non-corporate leader	Corporate leader
Uses moral arguments to describe goals	Uses plans and strategies
Informal style	Formal style
Personal style	Usually, impersonal style
Monitors performance directly	Monitors performance indirectly
Measures success by a range of factors, including relationships	Measures success according to outputs
Focused on developing potential of volunteers	Usually focused on developing competencies of followers
Takes all volunteers seriously	Some followers appear to be more valued than others
Equal access to leader	Leader protected by 'gate keeper'
Has explicit set of diverse and personal beliefs	Personal beliefs often implicit
Works collaboratively, building alliances across many organizations	Most working relationships limited to within the organization

I now want to tell a few stories to show some of the results of these differences in style in (leadership) and content (the work that is done). The stories are from the UK, the USA, and South Africa.

STORIES OF EXCEPTION

The UK – The Broadwater Farm Health Project (BWFHP)

Most people in the UK know Broadwater Farm as the place of the riot in the 1980s in which a policeman was killed. This was also my first knowledge of the existence of this housing estate. But Broadwater Farm is more than a newspaper headline.

It sits in the middle of the borough of Haringey in London, and houses several thousand people of varying nationalities, cultures, professions and ages. It also houses schemes to equip young people for employment, schemes which have an international reputation.

I first heard about the BWFHP project while working at the RHA which funded the health centre, opened on the Farm in 1995. My job included responsibility for developing user involvement in planning and delivering health services. The BWFHP was unique in that it was residents who, on finding out the extent of the poor health status of their community, had asked the local public health department for help in finding solutions. After this meeting, it was agreed to use residents' concerns about health needs on the estate to launch a health project.

The Project consisted of three programmes:

1. A community-focused needs assessment
2. A health promotion and information campaign
3. An estate-based community primary healthcare centre.

North East Thames Regional Health Authority awarded £525 000 for the third programme, which was completed and opened in November 1995. The project was a collaboration between the health authority, the local authority and Broadwater Farm residents, and more recently, the local community trust and the primary healthcare division of the local university. The leadership of the project resided with the residents' association, which consisted of the leaders of different groups in Broadwater Farm, and which coordinated the meetings to progress the project.

I attended a few of these meetings while based at the RHA and was struck by the determination of the residents to realize their dream of an on-site health centre. Their determination stemmed from knowing that, given the reluctance of many local GPs to take Broadwater Farm residents onto their register, only a service which centred on their needs would help to improve the health status of residents. To this end, recruitment of a GP to work at Broadwater Farm was begun.

In keeping with the health authority's stated aim of involving service users more closely in planning and delivering health services, residents were part of the selection process for the GP. At the first attempt, no appointment was made because no applicant met the key criterion – a focus on caring for the residents of Broadwater Farm. Residents were looking for a relationship with the GP, not just a transaction. They also wanted the GP to be accountable to residents for the care given.

Neither the Department of Health nor the health authority was particularly happy with residents helping to select their GP, but they did not give up and eventually selected a GP of their choice, and then selected someone else when that relationship broke down. Residents were also involved in the selection of a nurse to develop out-reach services.

During the time that the primary care centre was being built, another issue surfaced which tested the leadership of the project. The local authority unilaterally made changes in the design of the primary care centre. Part of the planning process used up about one-third of the total cost of £525 000, so the changes were inevitable. Residents understood the need for planning. What they did not understand was why the local authority had provided that particular in-house plan, when the private sector could offer a more competitive option? And why had they not consulted residents, as they had agreed, as one of the ground rules of the project? By breaking their word, the local authority had tampered with their dream. They had been treated with a lack of respect.

At stake was the issue of accountability. The resident's association knew they were accountable to all the residents on Broadwater Farm. To whom was the local authority accountable? And was this the way they treated their staff? But this hiccough did not stop the resident's association from continuing their daily role of overseeing the project and keeping all residents informed of progress. When the primary care centre opened in November 1995, it was a testament to leaders who had stayed focused, determined, and motivated enough to mobilize others to help the project succeed.

The BWFHP is a very local example of what can be achieved by people who want to change things. The leadership of the BWFHP was not nice and neat; in fact, at times it was chaotic and fractious. From what I saw of these leaders, they were going through the stages of group development. There was an overall leader in the group, who spent most of the time reminding others of the initial reasons the project was started. This person also secured funds for the development of the residents' association, and to evaluate the project.

Since the first meeting with the health authority, the BWFHP has developed into a community-based regeneration project. There are tentative plans to have an education centre based on Broadwater Farm, with links to the local university. Lecturers would deliver their courses on-site, and residents would be able to access all the courses offered by the university.

The BWFHP is led by people who are self-selected and who live with the issues on Broadwater Farm, and therefore have a continuity with the life of the project that is unusual in structured organizations. A bare majority of these leaders are women, another difference from structured organizations.

The project continues to grow, and may well form the nucleus of other initiatives in community participation.

South Africa – 'Bad men came'

This story was told to me by the person it happened to. The story teller is a nurse manager in a large hospital in the Kwa Zulu Natal province of South Africa. At the time of the related incident, there was continuing violence in that province. Many people were killed, or lost their homes and families.

One morning before daybreak, the nurse manager received a telephone call from one of the nurses who was due at work on the early shift. She was calling to say that she would not be at work that day because she could not get there. When asked why, she said 'Last night the bad men came. I had to run with my children to the bush and hide. I am there now'.

The response from the manager was immediate. She got dressed, got in her car and drove for miles to where her colleague was hiding, then took her and her children to a place of safety.

I think of this story often, especially since I read that NHS staff who report sick will be visited at home to check if their illness is legitimate. How many leaders in your organization know that rescuing and protecting followers from harm is part of their job? Remember 'tit for tat'? Non-corporate leaders believe in this totally. To put it another way, positively stroking people appears to be a vital part of the success of non-corporate leaders. In many structured organizations people get stroked only when someone wants something from them.

During apartheid, many nurses died when the bad men came. Many nurses also take leadership roles in their communities, sometimes against the wishes of some men who do not believe women should lead. In South Africa, there are many stories like the one above. Each attests to the endurance of the human spirit under the most extreme circumstances. At the centre of each is a leader who thought something, did something, and changed something.

USA – Women and children first

Earlier in this chapter, I talked about a non-profit healthcare agency I worked with. I want now to illustrate how non-corporate forms of leadership can generate dynamic change in communities.

The agency in question is called the Brooklyn Perinatal Network (BPN) (you will remember that I described its work in Chapter 2, when I related the story of Lynda Randolph). The BPN is based in Bedford-Stuyvesant, which has an inner-city's socio-economic and demographic profile – high unemployment, crime, poverty, inadequate and inappropriate health services. In spite of this, Bedford-Stuyvesant, probably the largest African-American community in the USA, is now seen as a model for community development; one result of this community's 30-year history of pro-active planning and collaborative working.

A significant aspect of Bedford's success in community regeneration has been the Bedford-Stuyvesant Conference, a 10-member task force which represents the major aspects of life in the community – economic development, youth, women and children, families, transportation, housing and crime. The creation of local school boards, the formation of the Coalition For Quality Education, the establishment of the Boys and Girls High School are all results of concerted community action. All this activity is led by local leaders, who have a dynamism which can be startling. They make things happen.

The focus of BPN's work is reducing the infant mortality rate (IMR) (in the UK, perinatal mortality rate) in the Bedford district. BPN is an incorporated agency and is required to develop plans for health and other issues affecting the community. The agency holds itself accountable to the local community, and depends on it for resources and strength. BPN has about 20 staff with expertise in health education, finance, administration and data analysis.

While BPN's major strategy is to identify and resolve issues about local service delivery, it also has a key role in regenerating the districts it serves. One district, Forte Greene, has as high IMRs as Bedford, but were not included in the project to reduce the overall statistics. After consulting with community leaders in Forte Greene, BPN sponsored a Neighbourhood Based Alliance (NBA) to enable Forte Greene to apply for funds to map gaps in healthcare provision.

The process of the application provided an insight into how powerful, non-corporate forms of leadership can be. In the space of 4 weeks, BPN:

- Coordinated a bidders' conference whereby community-based organizations who wanted to make a collaborate bid under the NBA met with a state official who gave detailed information about the application process.
- Resourced a series of meetings with the Forte Greene community groups who wanted to collaborate on a bid. The chair of the group was an experienced volunteer.
- Targeted a state Congressman to be present at a community 'speak-out', and convened a hearing at which constituents presented evidence of gaps in service provision and economic development. The Congressman explained, with mixed success, how the then healthcare reforms would improve the health of Forte Greene residents.
- Discovered and decided to mentor a young Forte Greener who wanted to improve garbage disposal in his building.

- Succeeded in getting Chase Manhattan Bank, a major employer in Brooklyn, to join the Fort Greene coalition.
- Coordinated the NBA application.

Although the application was not wholly successful, BPN had started a process which has since begun to improve the health of Forte Greene.

NHS – Some short stories

- The manager who started a new job, needed to get his office painted, and was told he would have to wait 3 months. So he painted it himself, the next day. This man always has a screwdriver to hand, just in case he finds something that needs to be repaired.
- The midwifery manager who threw an impromptu party at lunch time for staff who had given up lunch breaks over several weeks to get a new project off the ground. She used her own money.
- The chief executive who always wants to know how his fellow directors feel about the things they see and hear as they walk around their hospital. Which means they have to walk around their hospital.
- The training manager who, in planning staff training, wants to know why people in the organization come to work. He has discovered that many of his colleagues do not have an answer to this question.
- The midwife who offered me a roof over my head when I did not have one. I had worked with her for about three shifts.
- The university department head who always wanted to know what was your dream for next year. He knew his staff could do their technical jobs; he just needed to be sure that we did not lose ourselves while doing them.

You have your own stories of exceptional leaders who lead exceptional organizations. No memos, no waiting for the other shoe to drop, no waiting to see if someone else is going to take action. They get it done, through volunteers. We need more leaders like this in nursing, in the NHS, everywhere. But it would seem that they do not thrive in structured organizations. So, maybe we should create the environment for them to thrive inside these places – small units, with autonomy, with a focus on people and the bottom line.

We need to learn more about how they inspire, motivate and mobilize volunteers. The continued existence of the BWFHP, BPN, and others, strengthens my belief that non-corporate forms of leadership are key to achieving what we say we want from our leaders – people with ideas who can enable us to dream dreams and fulfil them.

Non-corporate leaders are not wishy-washy. They are skilled managers who expect that goals will be met and financial accountability maintained. But they are also exceptional leaders who value the relationship with volunteers highly. The more we become aware of this type of leader, the more we might be able to create in the workplace, that sense of community that is increasingly necessary for our well-being, and for organizational success.

There is a growing interest in alternative models of leadership. For example, Mawson talks about 'social entrepreneurs' (Mawson 1998), leaders who 'recognize that the knowledge and ideas of their staff are their most important resources'. Such leaders 'communicate their aims in moral terms'. Recently, the idea for a course on developing social entrepreneurs was launched by Michael Young (Lord Young), a great example of a non-corporate type of leader, whose ideas created the Open University and the Consumer Associations, among others.

NURSE LEADERS IN NON-CORPORATE SETTINGS

If nurses are to be successful leaders in settings where there are few formal leaders, then we need to learn how to lead volunteers. We need to create movements passionately committed to making change for the better. There are numerous projects and ideas rolling around health and social care that will feed and inspire the spirit of leaders and volunteers – equity, justice, mental health services, endemic racialism in employment and service delivery, poor quality service at the margins of care, lack of respect for each other, ramshackle environments, indifferent leadership, getting the best from people, and so on. But on closer inspection, the current priorities for health and social care are also instrumental – for example the private finance initiative (PFI), primary care groups (PCGs), clinical governance.

I find it difficult to get fired up about PFI or PCGs or any of the very big ideas for structural change to health and social care when I know of hospitals where you cannot get a glass to give a patient a drink of water. It is at the margins that passion can make a difference. Clinicians have often been accused of 'shroud waving' to prevent change from happening. But if under that shroud are the ideas that will create more organizations, wave away.

What non-corporate leaders show us is that people will volunteer to follow an idea which gives an opportunity to make things better. The idea does not have to be big, but it must enable volunteers to feel connected to something beyond themselves. For the foreseeable future, we have to engender this passion inside structured organizations, so be prepared for the consequences – frustration at the slow pace of change, impatience with the structure, territorial conflicts, increased visibility (making you easy to shoot down), exhaustion, and an initial lack of volunteers. Only you can decide if the prize – organizations which nurture and reward the human spirit – is worth the price.

Key learning points

- Non-corporate leaders have volunteers.

- Non-corporate leaders place a high value on their volunteers.

- Non-corporate leaders know that they are dependent on their volunteers.

- Non-corporate leaders are driven to get things NOW.

- Effective non-corporate leaders are also good managers.

REFERENCES

Blanchard K 1996 The one minute manager builds high performing teams. Harper Collins, London
De Pree M 1997 Leading without power: finding hope in serving community. Jossey-Bass, San Francisco
Fisher A, Martin J, Levering R, Moskowitz R 1998 The 100 best companies to work for in America. Fortune 12 January: 21–35
Mawson A 1998 The rise of the social entrepreneur. Journal of the Royal Society of Arts cxlv (5484), 1/4, 91–99

So what?

Process me this and process me that 205	Oops 206

Key words:

So what?

So what that leadership is a choice? So what that hindsight is a fun activity that should be reserved for rainy days? I have not always found it a particularly helpful aid to learning. What has been useful is forethought, which depends on self-knowledge and hubris-free consideration of the risks involved in any venture.

In this, I have not been nearly as successful as I would have liked. On the other hand, I am not easily upset or discouraged, and rarely take any insult (whether natural or manufactured) personally. That may be the result of another of the many lessons I learned from my mother – life is a test of your sense of humour.

As it is, personal success as a leader has been liberally interspersed with errors and mishaps, near-misses and near-catastrophes, none of which seemed funny at the time. The notion that somehow we can control the events we experience is fallacious. Chaos is the natural order, and leaders work with it, not against it. As a leader, you have to work with what you have, and try to bargain for the rest.

My first conscious experience of this was as a project manager employed to implement the nursing process in a women's health unit – not a job for anyone who likes an ordered existence.

PROCESS ME THIS AND PROCESS ME THAT

A simple enough task, you might think. After all, planning patient care is better than the 'adhocracy' that nurses had practised for so long. Well, read on; you might catch similarities between my experience and that of Charge Nurse Leo, presented earlier in the book.

My first mistake was not fully recognizing the power of inertia, and the generally conservative nature of human beings and professional groups. Neither did I give enough attention to the history between the various groups in the unit. At that time in my life, I was less tolerant than I am now of people who resisted change. One consequence of both these mistakes was to create hostility to the project, which reflected onto me.

I remember the frustration at not being able to secure the whole commitment of senior nurses, and the sense of injustice that 'they' were making 'my' project fail. It took me 3 months to notice that resistance was highest among the most experienced staff, who felt excluded from both the content and the process of the project. Since I do not believe in conspiracy as an explanation of why change fails (well, not all the time), I figured that resistance from this group was more than bloody-mindedness. That meant having to review, with their help, the original plans for the project, as well as the method for implementation.

Out went persuasion based on my position, substituted by building personal influence based on knowledge, empathy, and an increased ability to laugh at myself. Food also played a large part – it is nearly impossible to argue and fight when your mouth is full, *and* you are laughing.

But this was only the first part of the problem fixed. As the project proceeded, more obstacles emerged. Each had to be viewed individually, and as part of its contribution to improving the project. That had been my next mistake – thinking that there is only ever one problem, or one person causing the problem. Once I stopped playing this game, whatever problem presented was seen as one more way to learn about something, or someone. This does not mean that I was swayed by every disagreement that arose. No, I learned how to lead, and when to follow.

The project was successful in that it changed the way nursing care in the unit was viewed. The model of care we developed is still used, albeit in an abbreviated form. There were other spin-offs, including patient-held records, and integrated notes. One of the nicest things for any leader is to see, years later, the result of previous work, and know that your efforts have produced longterm benefits. But some of my experiences as a leader have had more pain and significantly less gain.

OOPS

Sacking people, or making them 'redundant', is no fun. Neither is depriving patients of much needed care. I have had to do both, and although the fault was not mine, that has not detracted from the niggling sense of doubt that maybe I did not do the right thing, or the sense of loss, even though I feel I did it right.

The sackings and removal of care resulted from loss of funding to an HIV/AIDS-related voluntary organization I led. For small voluntary sector providers, no funding means closure, often at very short notice. My involvement in this event has taught me much about the responsibilities, and pain, of leadership.

First, it was never our intention to close the agency. Re-structure and re-focus, yes. Close, no. That decision was driven by funders. Second, re-locating our vulnerable patients depended on having available resources in the community who could duplicate our work. We found the best there was. But to this day, I am not convinced that it was good enough, and I believe our clients got a rotten deal.

Third, I had to ensure that staff were not unnecessarily traumatized at losing their jobs with less than 3 weeks' notice. That meant being a source of information about available jobs, even before they were advertised, and providing references as quickly as possible. We did much better with our staff than with our clients. But there was also a responsibility to statutory bodies (for example the Charity Commission) to wind up the agency in an acceptable manner. To add to the adventure, we have had to remain extant in order to recoup funds embezzled from the agency in its early years before it was incorporated as a charity.

In the meantime, this twilight zone existence continues, and with it a sense of unfinished business, especially for our clients. And yet, my feeling of failure is more about me not seeing clearly enough how government policy on HIV and AIDS would affect the agency's work. The fact that the health authorities funding the agency might have misled us is irrelevant. I should have had more nous.

But even using foresight to guess accurately that funding for HIV and AIDS would move away from specialist agencies in preference for more local provision, the agency's continuing existence might have depended on another kind of change. The agency would have been different, altered in some way, but only in relation to the dimension in which it existed. Let me give an example – from *Star Trek*, of course.

In an episode of *Star Trek – The Next Generation*, Worf inadvertently triggers multiple universes, into which manifest the *Enterprise* – several hundred of them. Each of the starships are physically the same. But each crew is having its own experience, in its own universe, without knowing about the existence of its counterparts. In a similar way, the agency in this universe is the only one I know. There may well be several others which are thriving in another universe. If so, hindsight might help me access them and learn for next time. But all I had was the knowledge from here and now, and that is how I chose to respond.

Hindsight might make me feel better about the outcome (in other words, salve my conscience, or pass the blame onto others). But the me who has taken the action to close the agency, and the me who would be created by hindsight, are two different people. 'If only I had' is of little use after the event, especially if the intention is to use the knowledge to make it right next time. The next time you will be a different person, under different circumstances.

None of the experiences I have had as a leader has been the same. What has been constant is my attempt to remain consistent (not predictable). Consistency requires that some people are offended by some things that you do. But, as leaders, we aim to recruit volunteers, not a fan club.

While preparing this book, I have been more aware of leaders and leadership. It seems that every day, there are examples of failed leadership, or of a leader who fudged ethics, or emotion, or personal beliefs. Whether it is sexual harassment at Mitsubishi, Orangemen in Northern Ireland, managers of football teams, murder investigations, or the governance of the country, each day, leaders and leadership lose a little more credibility and become a little more like the monsters we have always suspected them to be.

But whose fault is it? What if these leaders we so despised acted honourably at all times, told us the truth at all times, and held us to account at all times? Would we have a better opinion of them? Probably, until such time when we decide that we have had enough of honour, and truth, and accountability. Leaders will never win popularity contests. The best they can do is follow the path they have mapped out, and hope to recruit the necessary volunteers. And yet, leaders need to win the battle against the apathy that stops all of us from becoming the leaders we can be. Restoring the balance between the Id, Ego and Superego would be a start. Ambition minus conscience and competence equals *Star Trek*'s Lt Commander Data without humour or a soul.

In 1998, the British National Health Service celebrated its 50th birthday. This is the UK organization about which I have the most knowledge. It is also the biggest organization in the world – 1.1 million staff, and a current annual budget of £42 billion. The conduct of leaders and leadership in an entity of that size and importance cannot be ignored. So far, the score between best practice on leadership and 'could do better' is moving imperceptibly in favour of the first. But the leadership of any group of people will only be as effective, appropriate, and successful as those who become the leaders and the volunteers.

Health service workers have many examples of failed leadership. What is less clear is whether this knowledge is helping us to get it more right and than the last time. With regard to nurses, we are still struggling against ingrained traditions of eating our young and undermining our leaders. Yearning for the old days of the all-conquering Matron will not enable us to develop the key political, social, and personal skills which we need to do leadership better.

The Royal College of Nursing (RCN) leadership programme is a start. Its intention is to produce a crop of clinical leaders who can influence both health policy and service planning and delivery. But, by itself, the RCN programme cannot possibly provide all the leaders nursing needs, nor should it. *Leadership is everybody's business.* It does not depend on who you are, but on what you do, and how you do it.

As the emphasis of the health service shifts back to the quality of care patients receive, the leadership needed will have its roots in clinical practice. That means that doctor, health visitor, nurse, midwife, occupational therapist, pharmacist, physiotherapist, podiatrist, psychologist, every other stripe of clinician will be required to set standards for clinical excellence. We will therefore be required to lead as never before. The buck will stop with us. If you doubt this scenario, reflect on Bristol. Only clinicians, working together, and with the courage to lead will prevent further calamities. Even then, mistakes will happen. But without leaders willing to lead, we may find ourselves taking part in the conspiracy that Bennis talks about.

Our conversation is over. I have enjoyed talking with you. I cannot force you to accept that you are a leader. The choice is yours. But it is so much better to have tested your mettle than not to have even entered the arena at all. Are you leader enough to try?

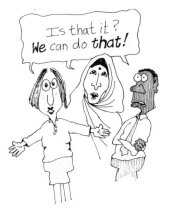

Key learning point

Leaders R us.

Further reading

Chapter 2

The books for this chapter are all easily available, except for Rosabeth Moss Kanter's, which needs to be ordered.

Ziggy Alexander and Audrey Dewjee re-discovered the life of Mary Seacole. Their edited book *The Wonderful Adventures of Mrs Seacole in Many Lands* is the second edition of Mrs Seacole's autobiography, first published in 1857.

Alexander Z, Dewjee A 1984 The wonderful adventures of Mrs Seacole in many lands, 2nd edn. Falling Water Press, Bristol

In Search of Excellence by Tom Peters and Robert Waterman was the first best seller on management. Peters and Waterman examined how (US) companies did management, and made management exciting. That many of the companies featured in the book have fallen on hard times since, does not detract from the sense of adventure which runs through the book.

Peters T, Waterman R 1995 In search of excellence. HarperCollins, London

The sequel to the above book, *A Passion for Excellence: The Leadership Difference* (co-authored with Nancy Peters) targeted leadership as the essence of longterm organizational success, and introduced that awful phrase, MBWA (Management by Wandering About).

Peters T, Waterman R, Peters N 1986 A passion for excellence: the leadership difference. Fontana, London

Rosabeth Moss Kanter is an acknowledged authority on organization development, especially gender issues. The central theme of her book, *Men and Women of the Corporation*, is the treatment of women in organizations.

Moss Kanter R 1977 Men and women of the corporation. Basic Books, New York

Max De Pree's *Leadership is an Art* is the story of how he has led his company, Herman Miller, a top-rated US furniture manufacturer. It is 148 pages of joy.

De Pree M 1989 Leadership is an art. Arrow, London

James Kouzes and Barry Posner wanted to find out how extraordinary things were done, and kept on being done in organizations. The result of their search is two books, both with the same title, and published 7 years apart – *The Leadership Challenge*. The 10 steps of leadership in Chapter 10 are based on some of the concepts in these books.

Kouzes J M, Posner B Z 1987 The leadership challenge: how to get extraordinary things done in organizations. Jossey-Bass, San Francisco

Kouzes J M, Posner B Z 1995 The leadership challenge: how to keep getting extraordinary things done in organizations. Jossey-Bass, San Francisco

The story of Aaron Feuerstein is told in more detail in an article by Thomas Teal – *Not a Fool, Not a Saint*. This is one of my favourite leader stories, partly because it is so hubric (that is my term for anything lacking in hubris).

Teal T 1996 Not a fool, not a saint. Fortune, 11 November: 111–113

Chapter 3

A general introduction to organization theory is *Writers on Organizations*, by D. S. Pugh and D. J. Hickson, which has been used as a text in the Open University's Certificate in Management Studies. Pugh and Hickson have also written *Organization Theory* (Penguin), which is a collection of some of the original articles by people such as Frederick Taylor.

Pugh D S, Hickson D J 1989 Writers on organizations. Penguin, London

Also useful is *Working in Organizations*, by Andrew Kakabadse, Ron Ludlow, and Susan Vinnicombe.

Kakabadse A, Ludlow R, Vinnicombe S 1988 Working in organizations. Penguin, London

Fred E. Fiedler's theory of contingency leadership was first published in *A Theory of Leadership Effectiveness*.

Fiedler F 1967 A theory of leadership effectiveness. McGraw-Hill, New York

P. Hersey and K. H. Blanchard set out their theory of leadership in 1969 in an article called *Life Cycle Theory of Leadership*.

Hersey P, Blanchard K B 1969 Life cycle theory of leadership. Training and Development Journal 23(5): 26–34d

Effective Leadership is a Local Government Management Board project on transformational leadership in the UK. It is authored by Professor Beverly Alimo-Metcalfe, and is available from the Local Government Management

Board (Telephone 0171 296 6600). Professor Alimo-Metcalfe writes on leadership issues generally, and gender issues in leadership in particular. For example, the article called *Leaders or Managers?*

Alimo-Metcalfe B 1996 Leaders or managers? Nursing Management 3(1): 22–24

Ways Women Lead, is a ground-breaking study by Judy B. Rosener.

Rosener J B 1990 Ways women lead. Harvard Business Review 68(6): 119–125

The article *Shatter the Glass Ceiling: Women May Make Better Managers*, by Bernard M. Bass and Bruce J. Avolio, reports on the survey which confirmed the results of Rosener's study.

Bass B M, Avolio B J 1994 Shatter the glass ceiling: women may make better managers. Human Resource Management 33(4): 549–560

John Kotter clarifies the difference between management and leadership in *A Force for Change: How Leadership Differs from Management.*

Kotter J 1990 A force for change: how leadership differs from management. Free Press, London

Kouzes J, Posner B 1987 The leadership challenge: how to get extraordinary things done in organizations. Jossey-Bass, San Francisco

How to Choose a Leadership Pattern, by R. Tannenbaum and W. H. Schmidt was published in the *Harvard Business Review*.

Tannenbaum R, Schmidt W H 1958 How to choose a leadership pattern. Harvard Business Review 36(2): 95–101

Leadership – Theory and Practice by Peter G. Northouse is an accessible collection of essays. Readable and well set out; there is a self-assessment questionnaire at the end of each chapter.

Northouse P G 1997 Leadership – theory and practice. Sage Publications, London

Chapter 4

Frederick Herzberg's theory of motivation is more fully discussed in *Writers on Organizations* by D. S. Pugh and D. J. Hickson, a collection of essays on the work of major thinkers on organizations. This book is the standard text for an Open University course on management, so always look for the latest edition.

Pugh D S, Hickson D J 1989 Writers on organizations, 4th edn. Penguin, London

The article by Patrick Butler on the NHS Chief Executive's forum (*It's Tough at the Top*) can be found in the *Health Service Journal*.

Butler P 1997 It's tough at the top. Health Service Journal, 6 November: 12–13

Rennie Fritchie's article, *How to Grow Leaders*, is also in the *Health Service Journal* and reports the findings of a survey on what the NHS needs to do best to develop and support chief executives. The one caveat I make about this article is its narrow focus on 'top leaders' like chief executives, especially as the people involved in the survey admitted that aspiring chief excutives are thin on the ground. That may be a good thing, if it enables us to see leadership as much wider than what happens at the top (or what is left of it) of an organization.

Fritchie R 1997 How to grow leaders. Health Service Journal, 6 November: 12–13

Larsen J 1988 Being powerful: talk into action. In: White R (ed) Political issues in nursing: past, present and future, vol 3. John Wiley, Chichester

Jeffery Pfeffer's *Managing with Power* is a dense (in the sense of many words) in-depth look at influence and politics in organizations. The book uses case studies to illustrate how personal power (or influence) has a much greater impact on organization than position. Another book on power, which takes a very radical view is *Power* by Steven Lukes. A mere 64 pages, including bibliography, it is still the best introduction to power. It focuses on invisible power relations, such as how societies suppress and avert conflict by not discussing certain issues, or ignoring them.

Pfeffer J 1992 Managing with power. Harvard Business School Press, Boston

Lukes S 1974 Power. Macmillan, London

David Seedhouse writes on healthcare issues. He discusses 'everday ethics' in *Ethics: The Heart of Health Care*.

Seedhouse D 1988 Ethics: the heart of health care. John Wiley, Chichester

The article *Leaders Learn to Heed the Voice Within*, by Stratford Sherman is still relevant 4 years on, and is especially relevant to the NHS in the light of Rennie Fritchie's article on the need for healthcare leaders to take time to reflect on what they do and how they do it (see reference above).

Sherman S 1994 Leaders learn to heed the voice within. Fortune 130: 4

The RCN Ward Leadership programme is described by Geraldine Cunningham in an article called *Ward Leadership*. The Ward Leadership programme is a product of the RCN's 'Nurses in Leadership' project, created in 1993. There is a selection of papers from a conference on the project, published as a supplement (*Nursing Standard*, 6 March 1996).

Cunningham G 1997 Ward leadership. Nursing Standard, 15 October: 20–25

If you do not want to buy a copy of *Emminent Victorians* by Lytton Strachey, the extracted part about Florence Nightingale is available as a 1996 Penguin 60s (one of the many such published as part of Penguin's 60th birthday in that year).

Chapter 5

Stephen Covey's best selling book, *The 7 Habits of Highly Effective People*, can seem simplistic at times. However, the Circle of Influence/Circle of Concern (pp 81–85) is a useful way of looking at how we can reduce our tendency to be paralyzed by events we cannot control. *The 7 Habits* is also a handy collection of truisms.

Covey S R 1994 The 7 habits of highly effective people. Simon and Schuster, London, pp 81–85

Beverly Alimo-Metcalfe's article, The F words can be found in the *Health Service Journal*. One of the things I like about Beverly's writings is the way the words she uses conjure up images. In this article the graphic image is of the NHS as a kind of deformed F (head bowed, cringing, trying to fold in on itself). Whereas, what we as healthcare leaders should strive for, is a service swinging its arms with confidence and energy.

Alimo-Metcalfe B 1993 The F words. Health Service Journal, July: 25

The article by Susan M. Barbieri, *Office Politics in the Nicer '90s*, is taken from a magazine called *Working Woman*, which is published in the USA. You can subscribe from the UK direct to the US distributor. The magazine focuses on professional and business women, emphasizing both personal, and organizational issues. It is worth a look. If you are interested, let me know and I can lend you a back copy as a taster.

Barbieri S 1993 Office politics in the nicer '90s. Working Woman, August: 34–37

I'M OK, You're OK, by Thomas Harris is available in Dillons, and other major booksellers. Eric Berne's *Games People Play* was the book that introduced the concepts now familiar as Life Positions. Also by Berne, and very useful, is *What Do You Say After You Say Hello?*

Harris T 1973 I'm OK, you're OK. Pan, London

Berne E 1968 Games people play. Penguin, London

If you plan to use Life Positions in training or for personal development, then *Transactional Analysis for Trainers,* by Julie Hay, is a very good introduction. The book is very accessible and full of activities.

Hay J 1996 Transactional analysis for trainers. Sherwood Publishing, Watford

Chapter 7

The Leadership Challenge by J. Konzes and B. Posner is a good read, if you ignore the initial sensation that the leaders studied seem too good to be true. Remember that scepticism is an option you choose.

Kouzes J, Posner B 1995 The leadership challenge: how to keep getting extraordinary things done in organizations. Jossey-Bass, San Francisco

Chapter 8

The *Harvard Business Review* is an excellent source of scholarly studies in leadership. Many of its articles are reproduced as classics, including *Teaching Smart People How To Learn* by Chris Argyris.

Argyris C 1991 Teaching smart people how to learn. Harvard Business Review 69(3): 99–109

Warren Bennis' book *Why Leaders Can't Lead: The Unconscious Conspiracy Continues* is widely available. He has written several books on leadership, all of which are worth more than a passing glance.

Bennis W 1989 Why leaders can't lead: the unconscious conspiracy continues. Jossey-Bass, San Francisco

The article *The Dark Side of Leadership,* by Jay Conger, was published in the *Organizational Dynamics* journal.

Conger J 1990 The dark side of leadership. Organizational Dynamics 19(2): 44–55

Linda Davidson's report on events at the Bristol Royal Infirmary, *Alarm Unheard or Unheeded,* is in the *Health Service Journal.*

Davidson L 1998 Alarm unheard or unheeded. Health Service Journal, 4 June: 14–15

Matthew Limb's report on the Tayside case is one of several such which have appeared in the *Health Services Journal* over the past few years.

Limb M 1998 Board games. Health Service Journal, 10 July: 9

The quote by Argyris and Schon is from David A. Kolb's chapter, 'The Process of Experiential Learning', in *Culture and Processes of Adult Learning.*

Kolb D A 1974 The process of experiential learning. In: Thorpe M, Edwards R, Hanson A (eds) Culture and processes of adult learning. Routreclge, London, p 147

Chapter 9

J. Sterling Livingston's article, *Pygmalion in Management*, appears in the *Harvard Business Review*.

Livingstone J S 1988 Pygmalion in management. Harvard Business Review 66(5): 121–130

The following articles, reports, and books focus specifically on transformational leadership.

Ways Women Lead is a ground-breaking study by Judy B. Rosener.

Rosener J B Ways women lead. Harvard Business review 68(6): 119–125

The article *Shatter the Glass Ceiling: Women May Make Better Managers*, by Bernard M. Bass and Bruce J. Avolio, reports on the survey which confirmed the results of Judy Rosener's study.

Bass B M, Avolio B J 1994 B J Shatter the glass ceiling: women may make better managers. Human Resource Management 33(4): 549–560

The article *The Transformational and Transactional Leadership of Men and Women*, by Bernard M. Bass and Bruce J. Avolio, gives results of a major study on the leadership styles of men and women in a variety of organizations, including hospitals.

Bass B M, Avolio B J 1996 The transformational and transactional leadership of men and women. Applied Psychology: An International Review 45(1): 5–34

See Chapter 3 Further Reading for the reference on the report on research on transformational leadership in the UK (the Local Government Board study authored by Professor Beverly Alimo-Metcalfe).

The first nine goals of successful introspection are fully explained in *Leaders Learn To Heed The Voice Within*, by Stratford Sherman.

Sherman S 1994 Leaders learn to heed the voice within. Fortune 110(4): 64–70

The Leadership Challenge: How to Keep Getting Extraordinary Things Done in Organizations (this is the 1995 study) by James M. Kouzes and Barry Z. Posner, is available at large bookstores.

Kouzes J M, Posner B M 1995 The leadership challenge: how to keep getting extraordinary things done in organizations. Jossey-Bass, San Francisco

There is an article called *The Leader's New Work: Building Learning Organizations*, based on *The Fifth Discipline: The Art and Practice of the Learning Organization*, a book by Peter M. Senge, which provides a helpful summary of the new roles, new skills, and new work of leaders. This article should be available through the library of most business schools.

Senge P M 1990 The fifth discipline: the art and practice of the learning organization. Doubleday, New York

Senge P 1990 The Leader's new work: building learning organizations. Sloan Management Review

The terms 'transformational leadership' and 'transactional leadership' were first articulated by James McGregor Burns in his book *Leadership*.

McGregor Burns J 1978 Leadership. HarperCollins, New York

Several articles on shared governance have been published in the health service press. The three mentioned in Chapter 9 are from nursing journals. In an article called *Give Up Your Power*, John Naish reports on Tim O'Grady's model of shared governance.

Naish J 1995 Give up your power. Nursing Management 2(2): 7

Sandra Legg and Marina Hennessy describe the shared governance approach being used by St. George's Hospital Trust, London in an article called *Fair Shares in Practice?*

Legg S, Hennesy M 1996 Fair shares in practice. Nursing Management 2: 6–7

The model of shared governance adopted by Pinderfield and Pontefract Hospitals NHS Trust is outlined by Dina Leifer in an article called *New Way of Leading*.

Leifer D 1997 New way of leading. Nursing Standard 11(51): 12

Political Issues in Nursing: Past, Present and Future, edited by Rosemary White, is still a good introduction to the politics of nursing.

White R 1988 Political issues in nursing: past, present and future, vol 3. John Wiley, Chichester

Chapter 11

For easy reference, the references in Chapter 11 are grouped alphabetically into four categories – general leadership, nursing leadership, non-corporate forms of leadership, and other. These articles and books are just a small sample of the current literature on leadership. Browse in any sizeable bookstores and make your own choices.

General leadership

Bass B M, Avolio B J 1989 Potential biases in leadership measures: how prototypes, leniency, and general satisfaction relate to ratings and rankings of transformational and transactional leadership construct. Educational and Psychological Measurement 49: 509–526

Bradford D L, Cohen A R 1984 Managing for excellence, Wiley, Chichester

DePree M 1997 Leading without power: finding hope in serving community. Jossey-Bass, San Francisco

Kotter J P 1990 A force for change: how leadership differs from management. The Free Press, London

Rosener J 1990 Ways women lead. Harvard Business Review, November–December: 119–125

Stewart R 1989 Leading in the NHS: A practical guide. Macmillan, London.

Wilkinson D Y 1992 Indigenous community health workers in the 1960s and beyond, in Braithwaite R L Taylor S E (eds) Health issues in the black community. Jossey-Bass, San Francisco

Leadership in nursing

All of these articles are easily available, except *Caring* magazine, and Ann-Marie Rafferty's report. If you are interested in either of these, contact me.

Antrobus S 1998 Political leadership in nursing. Nursing Management 5(4): 26–28

Bowman G 1997 Over managed. Nursing Standard 11(19): 24–25

Casey N 1995 The great quest for leadership. Nursing Standard 10(12–14): 49–52

Casey N 1996 Student nurses unable to provide leadership. Nursing Standard 11(8): 8

Cunningham G 1997 Ward leadership. Nursing Standard 12(4): 20–25

Cunningham G, Whitby E 1997 Power redistribution. Health Management, September: 14–15

Falco Scott F 1995 Getting to the Year 2000, Caring, October: 17–18

Girvin J 1996 Leadership and nursing: Part 1: history and politics. Nursing Management 3(1): 10–12

Greenwood A 1997 Leadership for change. Nursing Standard 11(19): 22–24

Keighley T 1996 Editorial. Nursing Management 2(9): 3

Malby R 1996 King's Fund ignites the lights. Nursing Management 2(8): 11–13

Nazarko L 1996 Home front Leadership. Nursing Management 3(1): 16–17

RCN Nursing Update, Unit 062 1995 Leadership in nursing: more than one way. Nursing Standard 13(10)

Rafferty A-M 1995 Political leadership in nursing: the role of nursing in health care reform. Final Harkness Report (Commonwealth Fund of New York). Unpublished

Sams D 1996 The development of leadership skills in clinical practice. Nursing Times 96(28): 37–39

Wedderburn Tate C 1996 Out of the trench: developing nurse leaders. Nursing Standard 10(24): supplement, 8–9 This supplement contains several articles on leadership which are selected papers from a conference on nursing leadership (Nursing: The Leading Edge of health care, December 8–9 1995, London.)

Wilk J, Talbert V 1996 A handshake with the future. Nursing Standard 10(48): 25–27

Non-corporate forms of leadership

The first article below is a report of a lecture given at the Royal Society of Arts, and is available on tape (telephone the Society's lectures office, 0171 930 5115, for further information). A book of the same name as the article is published by DEMOS (telephone 0171 353 4479 for more information).

Mawson A 1998 The rise of the social entrepreneur. Journal of the Royal Society of Arts cxlv(5485), 1/4, 91–99

Wedderburn Tate 1996 Different ways to make a difference. Nursing Standard 10(29): 20

Other

The first reference is the report of a Department of Health funded survey, and was widely distributed throughout the NHS. The penultimate reference reports on a study funded by the English National Board.

Beishon S, Satnam V, Hagell A. 1995 Nursing in a multi-ethnic NHS. Policy Studies Institute

Buchan J 1998 Your country needs you. Health Service Journal 108(5613): 22–25

Clark G 1996 On-line midwives. Nursing Times 92(3): 18–19

Gerrish K, Husband C, MacKenzie J 1996 Nursing for a multi-ethnic society. Open University Press

Goodman M 1998 Ethical issues in health care rationing. Nursing Management 29–33

Chapter 12

To date, Max De Pree has written four books, three concentrating on leadership. The two I have used in this chapter are *Leadership is an Art* and *Leading Without Power: Finding Hope in Serving Community*.

De Pree M 1989 Leadership is an art. Arrow, London

De Pree M 1997 Leading without power: finding hope in serving community. Jossey-Bass,

The stages of group dynamics were adapted from Kenneth Blanchard's *The One Minute Manager Builds High Performing Teams*. This book has great diagrams which link leadership styles to each stage of group development.

Blanchard K 1996 The one minute manager builds high performing teams. HarperCollins London

The 100 Best Companies to Work For in America was a lead article in *Fortune* magazine. This magazine is published weekly and is available in the bigger newsagents, like WH Smith. It can also be ordered, by subscription, or you can visit their Web site: http://fortune.com.

Fisher A, Martin J, Levering R, Moscowitz M 1998 The 100 best companies to work for in America. Fortune 12 January: 21–35

Reverend Andrew Mawson's article, *The Rise of the Social Entrepreneur*, appears in the *Journal of Royal Society of Arts*. See Chapter 11 Further Reading for reference.

Details of the Broadwater Farm Health Project are in the report of the 1993 Focus Group Report. If you want more information, call the health centre (0181 365 1022) or contact Margaret Lally, Director – Child & Adult Services, Haringey Healthcare Trust, 0181 442 6000.

Index